How to Love Someone with Cancer

A Supportive Guide to Caring and Connecting Through the Cancer Journey

Rachel J. Oles

Table of Contents

Chapter 1

<u>AN OVERVIEW OF CANCER</u>

How cancer originates

Cells are the basic units that make up the human body. Cells grow and divide to generate new cells as the body needs them. Usually, cells die because they are too old or damaged. Then, fresh cells take their place.

Cancer originates when genetic changes interfere with this ordered process. Cells start to expand uncontrollably. These cells may create a growth called a tumour. A tumour could be malignant or benign.

A cancerous tumour is malignant, meaning it can develop and spread to other parts of the body. A benign tumour suggests the tumour can grow but will not spread.

Some forms of cancer will not create a tumour. These include leukemias, most forms of lymphoma, and myeloma.

TYPES OF CANCER

Doctors classify cancer into categories based on where it begins. Four main kinds of cancer are:

Carcinomas: A carcinoma arises in the skin or the tissue that covers the surface of internal organs and glands. Carcinomas frequently produce solid tumours. They are the most frequent type of cancer. Examples of carcinomas include prostate cancer, breast cancer, lung cancer, and colorectal cancer.

Sarcomas: Sarcoma begins in the tissues that support and link the body. A sarcoma can develop in fat, muscles, nerves, tendons, joints, blood vessels, lymph vessels, cartilage, or bone.

<u>Leukemias:</u> Leukaemia is a cancer of the blood. Leukaemia occurs when healthy blood cells mutate and grow uncontrolled. The 4 basic forms of leukaemia are acute lymphocytic leukaemia, chronic lymphocytic leukaemia, acute myeloid leukaemia, and chronic myeloid leukaemia.

<u>Lymphomas:</u> Lymphoma is a cancer that begins in the lymphatic system. The lymphatic system is a network of arteries and glands that assist combat infection. There are 2 main kinds of lymphomas: Hodgkin lymphoma and non-Hodgkin lymphoma.

<u>HOW CANCER SPREADS</u>

As a cancerous tumour grows, the circulation or lymphatic system may transmit cancer cells to other regions of the body. During this phase, the cancer cells multiply and may grow into new tumours. This is known as metastasis.

One of the first sites cancer typically spreads is to the lymph nodes. Lymph nodes are tiny, bean-shaped structures that help fight infection. They are scattered in clusters in numerous parts of the body, such as the neck, groyne area, and under the arms.

Cancer may also travel through the circulation to distant sections of the body. These parts may include the bones, liver, lungs, or brain.

Even if the disease spreads, it is still named after the place where it began. For example, if breast cancer spreads to the lungs, it is called metastatic breast cancer, not lung cancer.

Often, a diagnosis begins when a person visits a doctor about an odd symptom. The doctor will chat with the person about his or her medical history and symptoms.
Then the doctor will undergo many tests to figure out the reason for these symptoms.

But many patients with cancer have no symptoms. For many persons, cancer is detected during a medical test for another issue or condition.

Sometimes a clinician finds cancer during a screening test in a healthy person. Examples of screening tests include colonoscopy, mammography, and a Pap test. A person may need supplementary tests to confirm or deny the result of the screening test.

For most cancers, a biopsy is the only approach to provide a definite diagnosis. A biopsy is the removal of a tiny sample of tissue for future examination. Learn more about making a diagnosis following a biopsy.

<u>CAUSES OF CANCER</u>

Cancer is a complicated set of disorders characterised by the uncontrolled development and spread of abnormal cells throughout the body. While the specific causes can vary based on the type of cancer and individual variables, various underlying elements play a part in the development of this difficult disease.

1. Genetic Factors:

- <u>Genetic mutations:</u> Inherited genetic mutations can boost the probability of having certain types of cancer. Mutations in certain genes, such as BRCA1 and BRCA2, are connected to breast and ovarian cancer.

- <u>Family history:</u> A family history of various malignancies can heighten an individual's vulnerability. However, most cancers occur in adults without a family history.

2. Environmental Exposures:

- <u>Carcinogens:</u> Exposure to carcinogens, substances that encourage the development of cancer, can occur through air, water, food, or working settings. Examples include tobacco smoke, asbestos, radon, and certain chemicals used in companies.

- <u>Radiation:</u> Ionising radiation, such as from excessive X-ray exposure or nuclear accidents, can damage DNA and boost the risk of cancer.

3. Lifestyle Choices:

- <u>Tobacco usage:</u> Smoking and tobacco use are leading drivers of various malignancies, including lung, mouth, throat, and bladder cancer.

- <u>Diet:</u> A diet high in processed foods, red and processed meats, and low in fruits and vegetables may boost cancer risk.

- <u>Alcohol intake:</u> Excessive alcohol usage is connected with an increased risk of developing numerous types of cancer, including liver, mouth, throat, and breast cancer.

- <u>Lack of physical activity:</u> Sedentary lifestyles promote obesity, which is related with an expanded risk of several types of cancer.

4. Chronic Infections and Inflammation:

- Some persistent infections are associated with increased cancer risk. Examples include human papillomavirus (HPV) and cervical cancer, hepatitis B and C viruses and liver cancer, and Helicobacter pylori and stomach cancer.
- <u>Chronic inflammation:</u> Long-term inflammation due to disorders like inflammatory bowel disease or chronic gastritis can cause cell damage and lead to cancer formation.

5. Hormones and Hormone Therapy:

- Hormones exert a vital role in cancer development. Hormone replacement medication, particularly oestrogen, and progesterone during menopause, can elevate the risk of breast and ovarian cancer.

- Hormones in oral contraceptives can modestly boost the incidence of breast and cervical cancer, but the overall risk is negligible.

6. Age and Genetics:

- Age is a key risk factor, as cancer becomes more common as people get older due to accumulated DNA damage over time.

- Inherited genetic alterations can enhance the risk of certain malignancies, however, they normally account for a tiny number of instances.

7. Unknown or Random Factors:

- In other circumstances, cancer develops without a clear known cause. Sporadic mutations that arise randomly during cell division can lead to cancer genesis.

The causes of cancer are complicated and often involve a combination of genetic, environmental, behavioural, and biological factors. While some risk factors are changeable through healthy lifestyle choices, others are beyond individual control.

Recognizing and understanding these reasons enable individuals to take preventive actions, seek frequent screenings, and make informed decisions to lower their risk of cancer and increase overall well-being.

<u>UNDERSTANDING THE STAGES OF CANCER</u>

Cancer is a complex disease that can advance through multiple phases, each marked by particular characteristics and implications for therapy and prognosis.

The staging system provides a standardised approach to characterise the amount of cancer within the body, helping healthcare practitioners select the best course of action. Here, we look into the phases of cancer, highlighting their relevance and how they influence treatment options and results.

1. **Stage 0: In Situ Cancer:** At this early stage, cancer cells are restricted to the layer of cells where they formed and have not invaded nearby tissues or spread to distant regions.

- Treatment often entails eliminating the aberrant cells, and the prognosis is generally favourable as the malignancy has not yet become invasive.

2. Stage I: Localised Cancer: Cancer is still localised to the organ or tissue where it originated and has not spread to surrounding lymph nodes or distant places.
- Surgery is often the initial treatment, with a good possibility of total removal and cure.

3. Stage II: Locally Advanced Cancer: Cancer has grown larger and may have started to infect neighbouring tissues or structures, but it has not moved to distant areas.
- Treatment may entail a mix of surgery, radiation therapy, and chemotherapy to target both the main tumour and any microscopic spread.

4. Stage III: Regional migrated: Cancer has infiltrated neighbouring lymph nodes or tissues and may have migrated to adjacent structures.

- Treatment frequently involves a mix of surgery, radiation therapy, and systemic treatments to target both the underlying tumour and potential metastasis.

5. Stage IV: Distant Metastasis: Cancer has spread to distant organs or tissues, commonly through the bloodstream or lymphatic system.
- Treatment may entail systemic medicines such as chemotherapy, targeted therapy, immunotherapy, and sometimes surgery or radiation to manage symptoms and prolong life.

6. Recurrent or Relapsed Cancer: Cancer that comes back after treatment or continues after an initial response is labelled recurrent or relapsed.

- Treatment options vary on variables such as the place of recurrence, past therapy, and the overall health of the patient.

Staging Methods: Staging involves a combination of clinical assessments, imaging tests (e.g., CT scans, MRI), biopsies, and sometimes surgical inquiry.

- The TNM method, which stands for Tumour size, lymph Node involvement, and Metastasis, is widely used to diagnose cancer stages. A numerical stage (0 to IV) is assigned based on the TNM data.

Staging supports treatment decisions by providing insights into the cancer's behaviour, extent, and possible spread.
- Earlier-stage cancers usually have higher treatment success rates and better overall results.

- Advanced stages may require more aggressive treatment alternatives and palliative care to manage symptoms and improve quality of life.

Dynamic Nature of Staging: Staging could shift over time due to the response to treatment, illness progression, or new findings.
- Regular monitoring and review of staging are required to adjust treatment regimens as needed.

Understanding the phases of cancer is vital in directing treatment options and generating fair expectations for results. Staging gives essential information about the cancer's extent, enabling healthcare practitioners to modify treatment approaches to each patient's particular needs.

Early detection, correct staging, and educated treatment options lead to better survival rates and enhanced quality of life for those experiencing the hardships of cancer.

<u>SYMPTOMS OF CANCER</u>

Cancer, a group of diseases characterised by the uncontrolled proliferation of aberrant cells, can present in a wide range of symptoms that vary based on the type of cancer, its location, stage, and individual features.

Early detection of cancer signals is crucial for quick diagnosis and efficient therapy. While symptoms can be broad and often overlap with other conditions, identifying common signals can aid in early discovery and improved results.

1. <u>Unexplained Weight Loss:</u> Sudden and unexplained weight loss, especially if severe, can be an early symptom of various diseases, such as lung, stomach, pancreatic, or esophageal cancer. Cancer cells consume a great amount of energy, resulting in weight loss even without significant changes in diet or physical activity.

2. <u>Fatigue and Weakness:</u> - Persistent fatigue and weakness that don't improve with rest can be symptomatic of several types of cancer. Cancer-related fatigue is generally more acute than usual tiredness and could interfere with routine activities.

3. <u>Modifications in Skin:</u> - Skin modifications, such as changes in moles, sores that don't heal, or new growths, can be indicators of skin cancer like melanoma. Yellowing of the skin and eyes (jaundice) might be an indicator of liver cancer.

4. <u>Persistent Pain:</u> - Chronic pain that doesn't subside and isn't related to a specific injury or condition should be evaluated. Pain can be an early or late symptom, depending on the type of cancer and its location.

5. <u>Prolonged Cough or Hoarseness:</u> - A prolonged cough, coughing up blood, or hoarseness might be early symptoms of lung

cancer or throat cancer. These symptoms should be explored, especially if they remain for weeks.

6. <u>Changes in Bowel or Bladder Habits:</u> - Changes in bowel habits, such as blood in the stool, persistent constipation, or diarrhoea, could be warning markers of colorectal or gastrointestinal malignancies. Similarly, blood in the urine or changes in bladder habits can imply bladder or kidney cancer.

7. <u>Difficulty Swallowing or chronic Indigestion:</u> - Difficulty swallowing or chronic indigestion can be symptomatic of esophageal, stomach, or throat cancers. These symptoms should not be dismissed, especially if they are new or increasing.

8. <u>Unexplained Bleeding:</u> - Unexplained bleeding or bruises, such as blood in the urine, bleeding between periods, or rectal bleeding, should be evaluated by a

healthcare specialist. These symptoms can be associated with several disorders, including bladder, ovarian, or colorectal cancer.

9. <u>Changes in Breast Tissue: -</u> Any changes in breast tissue, including lumps, dimpling, changes in nipple appearance, or discharge, should be promptly evaluated. These symptoms may signal breast cancer.

10. <u>Chronic Fever or Infections:</u> - Frequent or chronic infections and fever could imply a weaker immune system, possibly related to an underlying disease, such as leukaemia or lymphoma.

11. <u>Neurological Symptoms:</u> - Symptoms such as headaches, changes in vision, dizziness, or seizures can be connected to brain or nerve system malignancies.

Cancer symptoms are various and can be subtle, making early recognition and awareness vital. While these symptoms can overlap with other disorders, any persistent or inexplicable changes in the body should be properly investigated by a healthcare practitioner.

Maintaining regular health check-ups, identifying personal risk factors, and seeking medical attention for persistent or troubling symptoms can contribute to early detection and the best potential outcomes in the journey toward managing and treating cancer.

Chapter 2

DEBUNKING FAMOUS MISCONCEPTIONS ABOUT CANCER

Cancer, as a complicated and diverse group of diseases, has long been surrounded by misconceptions and myths that can lead to uncertainty, and anxiety, and even obstruct effective preventative and treatment efforts.

It's very vital to dispel these myths and present true facts to empower individuals with knowledge and foster better understanding. Here, we address some of the most renowned misunderstandings regarding cancer and present the genuine facts:

1. Misconception: Cancer is Always a Death Sentence:

- **Fact:** While a cancer diagnosis can be terrifying, not all malignancies are lethal. Advances in medical research, early detection, and individualised treatment options have greatly improved survival rates for many forms of cancer. Some malignancies are very treatable and curable when diagnosed at early stages.

2. Misconception: Cancer is infectious:

- **Fact:** Cancer is not infectious and cannot be spread from one person to another by touch, sharing utensils, or close contact. Cancer occurs from uncontrolled cell development within an individual's own body.

3. Misconception: "Superfoods" Can Cure Cancer:

- **Fact:** While keeping a balanced diet rich in fruits, vegetables, and nutrients is beneficial for overall health, there's no single "superfood" that can cure cancer. A balanced diet is crucial, but it's not a substitute for medical therapy.

4. Misconception: Cancer is Always Caused by Genetics:

- **<u>Fact:</u>** While genetic factors can contribute to an elevated risk of certain malignancies, they are not the sole cause. Environmental exposures, lifestyle behaviours, and other factors play a crucial role in cancer development.

5. Misconception: Mammograms Can Cause Breast Cancer:

- **<u>Fact:</u>** Mammograms, which are X-ray images of the breasts, expose humans to a very tiny level of radiation that is deemed safe. The benefits of early breast cancer diagnosis by mammography considerably outweigh the tiny radiation exposure.

6. Misconception: Antiperspirants and Bras Cause Breast Cancer:

- **Fact:** Scientific investigation has not identified a reasonable relationship between using antiperspirants or wearing bras and an increased risk of breast cancer. These claims lack reliable evidence.

7. Misconception: Only Smokers Get Lung Cancer:

- **Fact:** While smoking is a major risk factor for lung cancer, non-smokers can also develop the disease. Radon exposure, secondhand smoke, air pollution, and hereditary factors can lead to lung cancer in non-smokers.

8. Misconception: Sugar Feeds Cancer Cells:

- **Fact:** While cancer cells do eat glucose (sugar), there is no evidence to support the assumption that consuming sugar directly stimulates the growth of cancer. Moderation in sugar consumption is crucial for overall health but isn't a solitary cancer prevention strategy.

9. Misconception: Alternative Therapies Are Always Better Than Medical Treatments:

- **Fact:** Alternative therapies should not substitute evidence-based medical treatments. While complementary therapies like meditation or acupuncture might enhance well-being, unproven alternative treatments can be dangerous and postpone necessary medical action.

10. Misconception: Cancer Always Shows Obvious Signs:

- **Fact:** Some malignancies might be asymptomatic or present modest signs, especially in the early stages. Regular check-ups and screenings are vital for discovering malignancies before symptoms become apparent.

11. Misconception: All Tumours Are Cancerous:

- **Fact:** Not all tumours are cancerous. Tumours can be either benign (non-cancerous) or malignant (cancerous). Benign tumours do not invade neighbouring tissues or spread to other parts of the body, while malignant tumours have the potential to spread and become life-threatening.

12. Misconception: Cancer Can Be Cured by Cutting Out the Tumour:

- **Fact:** Surgical removal of a tumour is a frequent technique in cancer treatment, but it's often not sufficient on its own. Depending on the kind and stage of cancer, additional therapies including chemotherapy, radiation therapy, or targeted therapy may be necessary to remove leftover cancer cells and prevent recurrence.

13. Misconception: Pain Equals Cancer:

- **<u>Fact:</u>** While pain can be a symptom of cancer, it's not always symptomatic of the disease. Many different disorders can cause pain, and cancer may not produce discomfort until it reaches an advanced stage. Prompt assessment by a healthcare practitioner is crucial to establish the origin of discomfort.

14. Misconception: Cancer Only Affects Older Adults:

- **<u>Fact:</u>** Cancer can affect individuals of all ages, including children. While the risk of cancer does grow with age, cancer can occur at any stage of life owing to a mix of inherited, environmental, and lifestyle factors.

15. Misconception: You Can't Get Cancer if You're Fit and Healthy:

- **<u>Fact:</u>** While adopting a healthy lifestyle helps lower the risk of having cancer, it's not a guarantee against the disease. Genetics, environmental exposures, and other factors can play an impact in cancer development.

16. Misconception: All Cancer Treatments Cause Hair Loss:

- **Fact:** While chemotherapy is recognized for causing hair loss, not all cancer therapies have this side effect. Radiation therapy and targeted therapies, for example, may not induce hair loss.

17. Misconception: Cancer Can Be Prevented Totally:

- **Fact:** While certain lifestyle choices like avoiding tobacco, maintaining a healthy weight, and practising sun safety might lower the possibility of cancer, it's not practicable to entirely prevent the disease. Genetic factors and other influences also contribute to cancer risk.

18. Misconception: Cancer Will Always Return After Remission:

- **<u>Fact:</u>** Not all malignancies return after establishing remission. The likelihood of recurrence varies on the type of cancer, stage at diagnosis, treatment, and individual characteristics. Regular follow-up treatment is essential to monitor for recurrence.

19. Misconception: Cancer Research Progresses Rapidly:

- **<u>Fact:</u>** While enormous improvements have been accomplished in cancer research, progress might be delayed due to the intricacy of the disease. Research involves significant inquiry and assessment before new medicines are devised and approved.

20. Misconception: Natural or Herbal Remedies Are Always Safe:

- **<u>Fact:</u>** Natural or herbal medicines are not always safe and can interfere with cancer therapies or drugs. It's vital to discuss with healthcare doctors before introducing alternative medicines into a cancer treatment approach.

Debunking these assumptions about cancer is vital to convey real knowledge, lessen worry, and empower individuals to make informed decisions about their health.

By eliminating misunderstandings and fostering greater awareness about cancer, society may collectively work towards early identification, successful treatment, and increased care for individuals and families affected by this challenging disease.

Chapter 3

UNDERSTANDING THE PROCESS OF CANCER DIAGNOSIS

The diagnosis of cancer is a pivotal event that heralds the beginning of a journey toward understanding, treatment, and management.

Diagnosing cancer includes a rigorous and systematic process that incorporates clinical assessments, medical imaging, laboratory tests, and generally biopsy to determine the presence, nature, stage, and features of the condition.

Let's analyse the whole procedure of diagnosing cancer and the strategies applied to offer precise insights.

1. Clinical Evaluation: - A healthcare practitioner begins the diagnostic process by conducting a full medical history and physical examination. Symptoms, medical history, family history, and lifestyle variables are taken into consideration.

2. Medical visualising: - Imaging techniques such as X-rays, CT scans, MRI, ultrasound, and PET scans play a crucial role in visualising interior structures. These photographs assist in identifying abnormal growths, tumours, or worrisome locations that require extra examination.

3. Laboratory testing: - Blood testing can provide considerable information about the body's health and function. Elevated amounts of specific markers or substances can imply the occurrence of cancer or other medical conditions.

4. Biopsy: - A biopsy entails the removal of a tiny sample of tissue for examination under a microscope. Different sorts of biopsies include fine-needle aspiration, core biopsy, surgical biopsy, and endoscopic biopsy.

- The biopsy gives definitive confirmation of cancer, determines the type of cancer, and helps assess aspects such as cell type, aggressiveness, and presence of certain biomarkers.

5. Pathology study: - The collected tissue sample is transported to a pathology laboratory, where it undergoes detailed analysis by a pathologist. The pathologist evaluates the cells and tissues to establish the type of aberrant growth and offers vital information for diagnosis.

6. Molecular Testing: - Molecular testing analyses the genetic and molecular properties of cancer cells. This information helps guide therapy options and identify specific mutations or genetic variables that can influence treatment response.

7. Staging: - Staging determines the extent of cancer throughout the body and helps anticipate its behaviour. Staging involves clinical tests, imaging testing, and sometimes surgery to assess the size of the tumour, lymph node involvement, and potential metastasis to other organs.

8. Multidisciplinary Review: - After acquiring all diagnostic information, a multidisciplinary team of medical professionals, including oncologists, radiologists, pathologists, and surgeons, assess the data and cooperatively offer the ideal treatment plan.

9. Second Opinion: - Seeking a second opinion from another knowledgeable healthcare expert is a key step in validating accurate diagnosis and exploring various treatment choices.

10. Emotional Support: - A cancer diagnosis can be emotionally upsetting. Healthcare providers regularly connect patients with support resources, including counsellors, social workers, and patient advocacy groups.

11. Imaging Techniques for Cancer Diagnosis: - **X-rays:** Used to detect abnormalities in bones and some soft tissues.
- <u>Computed Tomography (CT) Scan:</u> Provides complete cross-sectional images of the body, aiding in finding malignancies and assessing their size and spread.

- <u>Magnetic Resonance Imaging (MRI):</u> Utilises magnetic fields and radio waves to generate detailed images of inner structures, helping in diagnosing malignancies and their features.

- <u>Ultrasound:</u> Uses sound waves to visualise organs and tissues and can assist guide biopsies or other procedures.

- <u>Positron Emission Tomography (PET) Scan:</u> Utilises a radioactive tracer to target areas of high metabolic activity, helpful in locating cancer cells.

12. Blood and Laboratory Tests: - Complete Blood Count (CBC): Measures several components of the blood, which can show abnormalities caused by cancer or its treatment.
- <u>Tumour Markers:</u> Certain substances created by cancer cells or the body in reaction to cancer can be discovered in the blood. Examples include PSA for prostate cancer and CA-125 for ovarian cancer.

- <u>Biological Tests:</u> Assess the function of specific organs impacted by cancer, like liver and kidney function tests.

13. Molecular and Genetic Testing:

- <u>DNA Sequencing:</u> Analyses the genetic material of cancer cells to uncover specific mutations or genetic abnormalities that can guide targeted therapy.

- <u>Gene Expression Profiling:</u> Measures the activity of particular genes to anticipate how aggressive a tumour may be and personalise treatment approaches.

14. Liquid Biopsies: - A non-invasive treatment that involves testing components like DNA, RNA, or proteins in the blood to find cancer cells or genetic abnormalities.

15. PET-Guided Biopsies: - Combines PET imaging with biopsies, allowing precision targeting of problematic regions for more reliable sample collection.

16. Interventional Radiology Procedures: - Techniques include fine-needle aspiration, core needle biopsy, and ultrasound-guided biopsies allowing sampling of tissues utilising minimally invasive procedures.

17. Biobanking and Research: - Tissue samples taken during biopsies are often preserved in biobanks for future research, contributing in understanding cancer development, progression, and treatment responses.

18. Importance of Accurate Diagnosis: - An accurate diagnosis informs treatment decisions, enabling healthcare providers to choose the most effective drugs according to the type and stage of cancer.
- Accurate staging and diagnosis helps foretell prognosis, aiding patients in understanding their disease's expected course and results.

19. Emotional Impact: - The diagnostic process can be emotionally distressing. Patients often endure worry, fear, and uncertainty.
- Access to emotional support, therapy, and patient support groups is crucial during this phase.

Diagnosing cancer demands a comprehensive method that draws upon various medical disciplines and current technologies.

The combination of clinical evaluations, imaging, laboratory testing, biopsies, and molecular analysis provides a thorough picture of the disease's nature, extent, and characteristics.

Accurate diagnosis is the cornerstone of good treatment planning, enabling healthcare practitioners to devise methods that offer the best odds of successful results while supporting patients emotionally throughout their cancer journey.

Chapter 4

<u>NAVIGATING THE EMOTIONAL ROLLERCOASTER OF CANCER</u>

A cancer diagnosis is a life-altering event that sets in action a tough emotional journey for both the patient and their loved ones.

The emotional rollercoaster is described by a range of intense sentiments that might alter over time, from shock and panic to hope and resilience.

1. Shock and Denial:
- The initial reaction to a cancer diagnosis typically involves shock and disbelief. It can be difficult to understand the weight of the news, leading to a temporary state of denial as individuals try to come to grips with the reality of their position.

2. Fear and Anxiety:

- Fear of the unknown, uncertainty about the future, and worries about treatment, prognosis, and potential pain can generate overwhelming anxiety. The dread of loss and change can also evoke heightened emotional responses.

3. Anger and Frustration:

- Patients and loved ones could perceive rage focused towards the ailment, fate, or even healthcare staff. Feelings of impotence and dissatisfaction could come from the impression of losing control over one's life.

4. Sadness and Grief:

- A cancer diagnosis frequently brings a sense of loss, not only of health but also of the life one has planned. Patients and loved ones may grieve for the life they envisioned and the potential influence on relationships, profession, and future ambitions.

5. Isolation & Loneliness:

- Despite the presence of support networks, both patients and loved ones sometimes feel alienated owing to the unique problems cancer brings. Feelings of loneliness can stem from difficulty communicating about the sickness or the sensation of not being understood.

6. Hope & Optimism:

- Amidst the challenges, many individuals find moments of optimism and happiness. Medical discoveries, extraordinary stories of survival, and the ongoing support of loved ones can offer optimism in the midst of sorrow.

7. Uncertainty and Anticipatory Grief:

- The ambiguity around treatment outcomes and prognosis can rise to anticipatory grief, as individuals regret projected future losses. This complex emotional state can impair decision-making and general well-being.

8. Role Reversal and Caregiver Stress:

- Loved ones who take on the task of caretakers may experience high levels of stress, tiredness, and emotional strain. The reversal of roles can be emotionally draining as caregivers navigate their own sentiments while aiding the sick.

9. Resilience and Growth:

- Over time, some individuals gain strength and resilience in combating cancer. They learn to adjust to new situations, have a better respect for life, and develop a heightened feeling of thankfulness.

10. Communication Challenges:

- Open and honest communication is vital, but discussing cancer may be tough for both patients and loved ones. Addressing concerns, fears, and hopes is crucial for emotional well-being.

11. Seeking Support:

- Both patients and loved ones benefit from getting emotional help. Support groups, counselling, and therapy can give a secure environment to vent concerns and connect with others suffering similar challenges.

12. Coping Mechanisms:

- Individuals employ unique coping techniques to overcome the emotional rollercoaster. Some find solace in creative hobbies like art or writing, while others turn to mindfulness, meditation, or exercise to relieve stress and anxiety.

13. Impact on Relationships:

- Cancer can strain relationships, as communication habits vary and emotions run high. It's usual for patients and loved ones to confront misunderstandings, disagreements, or a sensation of isolation.

14. Balancing Positivity and Realism:

- Striking a balance between having an optimistic view and being realistic about the hurdles ahead is a tough job. Both patients and loved ones need to process emotions while being aware about treatment possibilities.

15. The Duality of Strength and Vulnerability:

- The cancer journey exposes the duality of strength and frailty. Patients often draw on their inner fortitude to accept treatments, while also acknowledging moments of vulnerability when they need help.

16. The Role of Communication:

- Open and honest communication between patients and loved ones is crucial. Sharing fears, hopes, and concerns helps develop an environment of understanding and connection.

17. Addressing Unresolved Issues:

- Cancer diagnosis can bring unresolved issues to the surface. Patients and loved ones may address previous issues or unresolved emotions as they face the challenges of the disease.

18. Shifting Priorities and Perspectives:

- The emotional rollercoaster of disease often leads to a shift in priorities and perspectives. Individuals may reconsider their objectives, relationships, and what is genuinely important in life.

19. Celebrating Small Victories:

- Every step forward, be it a successful therapy, a pain-free day, or a favourable test result, becomes a cause for celebration. Recognizing these minor victories can increase morale.

20. Grief and Loss:

- Grief is not confined to the loss of life; it can include a wide range of losses, including physical capabilities, employment aspirations, and a sense of normalcy. Both patients and loved ones may face waves of anguish throughout the trip.

21. Long-Term Emotional Impact:

- Even after therapy or remission, the mental burden of cancer endures. Fear of recurrence, adjusting to a "new normal," and managing ongoing physical and mental ramifications could continue to impair sentiments.

22. Building Resilience Together:

- The emotional rollercoaster impacts not just the individual but also their entire support network. Loved ones have a critical role in providing comfort, and understanding, and helping suffering acquire resilience.

The emotional rollercoaster of cancer is a shared experience that affects both sufferers and their loved ones. Navigating this journey demands patience, kindness, and a deep grasp of the subtleties each individual feels.

By admitting and expressing feelings honestly, finding support, and building a feeling of unity, patients and their loved ones can work together to weather the hurdles and find strength in their shared journey through the highs and lows of cancer diagnosis and treatment.

Chapter 5

SUPPORTING A LOVED ONE WITH CANCER

When a loved one receives a cancer diagnosis, delivering emotional support becomes crucial. Being present for them in meaningful ways, and actively listening to their worries, hopes, and concerns, can make a huge impact on their journey towards healing and coping.

Here, we cover practical techniques to listen and provide emotional support during this trying time.

1. Be Fully Present:
- When spending time with your loved one, focus on them and their emotions. Put aside distractions and offer them your undivided attention.

2. Create a Safe Space:

- Establish an environment where youngsters feel safe expressing their feelings without judgement. Let them know that their emotions are valid.

3. Listen Actively:

- Actively listen by delivering your whole attention, keeping eye contact, and nodding to show you're engaged. This encourages open discourse.

4. Avoid Offering Solutions Immediately:

- Often, your loved one needs to release their emotions without receiving rapid solutions. Instead of offering advice, acknowledge their feelings by mentioning something like, "I understand this must be really difficult for you."

5. Reflect and Validate Emotions:

- Reflect their emotions back to them to signal that you understand. Phrases such as,

"It sounds like you're feeling..." might express your empathy.

6. Use Open-Ended Questions:
- Instead of asking yes-or-no questions, utilise open-ended questions to enable people to share their thoughts and feelings more fully.

7. Practise Non-Judgmental Listening:
- Avoid interrupting, criticising, or expressing your perspective unless they ask for it. Sometimes, all they need is a listening ear.

8. Show Empathy:
- Put yourself in their situation and offer genuine empathy. Saying words such as, "I can't imagine how hard this must be for you" indicates your understanding.

9. Respect Their Silence:

- Silence may be powerful. If your loved one is quiet, it's fine to be quiet too, providing them space to internalise their feelings.

10. Offer Physical Comfort:

- A simple touch, a hug, or simply holding their hand can bring comfort and reassurance.

11. Keep Their Preferences in Mind:

- Some people choose to communicate openly about their diagnosis, while others may prefer not to discuss it. Respect their interests and boundaries.

12. Provide Practical Support:

- Offer support with routine duties, transportation to appointments, and practical chores. This might reduce tension and offer your support.

13. Avoid Minimising Their Feelings:

- Avoid phrases such as, "Don't worry, everything will be fine." Instead, acknowledge their sentiments and fears without downplaying them.

14. Be Patient:

- Understand that emotions can fluctuate. Be patient and encourage your loved one to express themselves at their own speed.

15. Offer to Accompany Them:

- Attending doctor's appointments or treatments with your loved one could bring emotional comfort and make them feel less alone.

16. Share Positive Moments:

- Engage in activities that offer joy and laughter. Sharing joyful events might enhance their emotions and provide a relief from cancer-related anxiety.

17. Connect Them to Resources:
- Provide information on support groups, counselling programs, or online forums where they can interact with others who are going through similar circumstances.

18. Check-In Regularly:
- Regularly reach out to see how they're doing. A simple text message or call can mean a lot and convey that you care.

19. Respect Their Privacy:
- Respect their desire for privacy and their decision to share their diagnosis to others. Ask permission before disclosing their health with others.

20. Remember Self-Care:
- Caring for a loved one with cancer can be emotionally draining. Remember to prioritise your own self-care to maintain your own well-being.

21. Educate Yourself:

- Take the initiative to study about their unique type of cancer, treatment possibilities, and any adverse effects. This insight can help you better comprehend what they're going through and provide informed assistance.

22. Be a Source of Normalcy:

- While cancer might bring multiple changes, attempt to preserve a sense of normalcy in your interactions. Continue to engage in activities you both enjoy to provide moments of escape from the trials.

23. Express Your Love and Support:

- Don't overlook the importance of expressing your love and support verbally. Let them know that you're there for them and that they can count on you whenever required.

24. Practice Patience and Flexibility:

- Emotions can be unstable during this period. Practise patience and flexibility as their emotional demands may fluctuate from day to day.

25. Encourage Professional Support:

- Suggest the thought of seeking professional emotional help if you feel that their emotions are becoming overwhelming. Therapy or counselling could provide extra coping methods.

26. Be a Good Listener for Their Loved Ones:

- If your loved one wishes to discuss their feelings regarding their family members or friends, provide a sympathetic ear without judgement.

27. Address Your Own Emotions:

- Supporting someone with cancer can be emotionally tough. It's vital to handle your own feelings and seek your own aid if needed.

28. Provide Distraction and Enjoyment:

- Plan activities that can deliver a nice respite from the problems of cancer. Engaging in hobbies or spending quality time together can enhance spirits.

29. Celebrate Milestones:

- Celebrate not only treatment milestones but also personal triumphs, whether they're connected to health benefits or emotional breakthroughs.

30. Recognize Your Limits:

- While you want to be there for your loved one, understand your own limits. It's fine to ask for help or take breaks when needed.

31. Show Unconditional Love:

- Unconditional love implies being present regardless of the circumstances. Assure your loved one that your support won't decrease.

32. Acknowledge Their Strength:

- Recognize and honour their resilience and courage. Let them know that you're inspired by their strength.

33. Be a Source of Hope:

- Offer hope and optimism when appropriate. Sharing experiences of survival or recovery could bring encouragement.

34. Maintain Open Communication:

- Keep the channels of communication open. Ask how they're feeling and what they need, and communicate your own thoughts as well.

35. Adapt to Changing Needs:

- As their emotional needs develop during the cancer experience, be ready to adapt your approach to providing the support they require.

Supporting a loved one through their cancer journey involves compassion, empathy, and a commitment to being there for them emotionally.

By actively listening, offering practical help, and being a pillar of support, you may play a significant part in supporting them through the emotional challenges that come with the diagnosis and treatment of cancer.

Your steady presence and understanding can offer them the courage they need to face each day with hope and tenacity.

Chapter 6

<u>PRACTICAL WAYS TO HELP A LOVED ONE WITH CANCER</u>

When a loved one is facing a cancer diagnosis, giving practical support can have a tremendous impact on their well-being.

From doing daily responsibilities to offering support at medical appointments, your efforts can alleviate stress and allow them to focus on their treatment and recovery. Here, we dig into numerous ways to offer practical aid that might make a major impact in their route.

1. Meal Preparation:
- Preparing healthful meals or organising a food train helps relieve the stress of cooking for the sick and their caretakers.

2. Grocery Shopping:
- Offer to shop for meals and deliver it to their home. Ensure you're aware of any dietary constraints or preferences.

3. Household Chores:
- Assist with household duties including cleaning, laundry, and organising. These modest acts might help maintain a comfortable environment.

4. Childcare and Pet Care:
- If they have children or pets, offering to take care of them can give the patient much-needed relaxation.

5. Transportation:
- Drive them to medical appointments, treatments, or support group meetings. Ensure they have a reliable mode of transportation.

6. Appointment Coordination:
- Help arrange and keep track of their medical appointments, treatment plans, and follow-up visits.

7. Medication Management:
- Assist with arranging their meds, ensuring they're taking them as directed, and renewing prescriptions as needed.

8. Emotional Support:
- Be a listening ear and a source of solace. Offer emotional support through phone calls, texts, and in-person visits.

9. Accompany to Appointments:
- Attend medical visits with them to provide company, take notes, and offer emotional support.

10. Communicating with Healthcare Providers:

- With their consent, help interact with healthcare providers to address any questions or concerns they might have.

11. Help with Paperwork:

- Assist with medical documentation, insurance claims, and other paperwork that could be onerous during treatment.

12. Financial Assistance:

- Offer to help with financial tasks, such as paying bills, managing insurance claims, and discovering available resources.

13. Technology Support:

- Help them set up gadgets for virtual appointments, connect with support groups online, or stay in touch with loved ones.

14. Provide Entertainment:
- Offer books, journals, puzzles, or streaming subscriptions to provide entertainment during downtime.

15. Arrange Visits from Friends and Family:
- Coordinate visits from friends and family members who want to lend their support.

16. Help Create a Comfortable Space:
- Assist in establishing a peaceful and relaxing area for the patient to rest and recover.

17. Gift Cards and Care Packages:
- Provide gift vouchers for restaurants, grocery stores, or leisure services, or assemble care packages to raise their spirits.

18. Assist with Personal Care:
- Offer support with personal grooming, bathing, and dressing if needed.

19. Research Treatment Options:

- aid in studying therapy alternatives, clinical studies, and alternative therapies that could aid them.

20. Celebrate Milestones:

- Mark treatment milestones, birthdays, and other occasions with thoughtful gestures to enhance their spirits.

21. Respite Care:

- Offer to provide respite care, allowing the primary caregiver an opportunity to rest and revitalise. This can substantially relieve the caregiver's mental and physical stress.

22. Provide Reliable Information:

- Research trustworthy sources of information regarding their specific type of cancer, treatment possibilities, and anticipated side effects. Share this knowledge with them to empower intelligent decision-making.

23. Assist with Technology:

- Help them set up video calls to stay connected with friends and family who may not be able to visit in person.

24. Organise Support Network:

- Coordinate with friends, family, and neighbours to establish a support network that can assist with varied chores, providing a well-rounded support system.

25. Assist with Mobility Aids:

- If needed, support them to arrange for and use mobility devices such as crutches, wheelchairs, or house adjustments for safety.

26. Home Maintenance:

- Offer to maintain their yard, garden, or outside spaces to generate a welcoming and tranquil environment.

27. Educational Resources:

- Gather instructional resources covering their diagnosis, treatment alternatives, and undesirable effects. This can help individuals understand and control their disease more successfully.

28. Provide Relaxation Techniques:

- Share relaxation strategies such as meditation, deep breathing, or light motions to assist reduce stress and promote well-being.

29. Create a Care Calendar:

- Use internet tools to establish a care calendar where friends and family may sign up for specific tasks, providing a consistent flow of support.

30. Encourage Hobbies and Activities:

- Help them discover hobbies, activities, or interests they like as a positive distraction from the burdens of disease.

31. Respect Their Wishes:

- Respect their decisions and preferences when offering support. Some days, they might choose to be more autonomous, but on others, they may prefer extra aid.

32. Provide Company:

- Spend significant time with your loved one, engaging in activities they enjoy or simply providing companionship.

33. Arrange Entertainment:

- Arrange for entertainment like movie evenings, music, or virtual events that might help enhance their mood.

34. Celebrate Small Achievements:

- Acknowledge their improvement and appreciate tiny wins, whether it's completing a treatment cycle or having reduced discomfort.

35. Be Patient and Flexible:

- Understand that their requests may fluctuate from day to day. Be flexible and alter your help as required.

Practical aid is a practical method to demonstrate your love and support for a cancer sufferer. By taking care of everyday activities, coordinating appointments, and lending a helping hand, you may alleviate their stress and bring a sense of comfort during a hard time.

Your attentive efforts can boost their quality of life, allowing them to focus on their health and recovery with confidence and hope.

Chapter 7

MAINTAINING INTIMACY AND EMOTIONAL CONNECTION WHEN A LOVED ONE HAS CANCER

Cancer can have a major effect on relationships, particularly the emotional and personal link between couples. Coping with the sufferings of cancer while retaining intimacy involves understanding, communication, and mutual support.

Here, we address strategies to sustain emotional connectedness and deepen closeness throughout this trying period.

1. Open Communication:
- Honest and honest communication is key. Both partners should share their feelings, anxieties, and concerns to sustain an emotional connection.

2. Active Listening:
- Actively listen to each other without judgement, letting the other person share their emotions and opinions.

3. Empathy and Understanding:
- Cultivate empathy by placing yourself in your partner's position. Understand their perspective and comprehend their sentiments.

4. Shared Decision-Making:
- Involve your partner in medical decisions and treatment plans to make them feel valued and involved.

5. Normalising Feelings:
- Acknowledge that it's normal to feel a range of emotions throughout this period. Validate each other's feelings and reactions.

6. Quality Time:

- Spend quality time together, engaging in activities that you both enjoy. Create positive memories amidst the challenges.

7. Physical Affection:

- Express physical affection through hugs, handholding, or gentle touches to reinforce your emotional relationship.

8. Intimacy Beyond Physicality:

- Understand that connection goes beyond physical contact. Emotional connection, trust, and understanding are equally vital.

9. Shared Goals and Plans:

- Set shared goals for the future, whether short-term or long-term, to create a sense of purpose and hope.

10. Supportive Environment:

- Foster a supportive environment where both partners feel confident expressing themselves without fear of condemnation.

11. Seek Professional Help:

- Consider couples counselling or therapy to manage challenges together and establish efficient communication strategies.

12. Express Gratitude:

- Express appreciation for each other's support, gestures, and efforts to maintain the emotional connection.

13. Maintain Independence:

- While supporting your partner, you preserve your identity and independence. This might deepen the friendship.

14. Laughter and Joy:

- Find moments of delight and laughter together. Laughter can be a good approach for coping.

15. Celebrate Milestones:
- Celebrate both tiny and huge victories to remind yourselves of the progress you're making together.

16. Nurture Self-Care:
- Caring for oneself is vital to be emotionally present for your companion. Prioritise self-care routines.

17. Patience and Flexibility:
- Be tolerant of each other's emotional fluctuations and adapt to changes in routines and dynamics.

18. Share Responsibilities:
- Divide work and duties to prevent one partner from feeling overwhelmed.

19. Explore Intimacy Education:
- Look into resources like books, workshops, or support groups that focus on preserving closeness during health challenges.

20. Focus on Love:

- Remind each other of your love and commitment. Celebrate the strength of your relationship in conquering hardship.

21. Create Rituals:

- Establish important rituals or routines that provide a sense of stability and predictability in your relationship.

22. Express Love and Gratitude:

- Regularly express your love and gratitude for your partner's constant support and presence.

23. Celebrate Small Wins:

- Celebrate even the simplest victories, reminding yourselves of the resilience you share.

24. Share Dreams and Aspirations:

- Continue sharing your dreams, aspirations, and plans to retain a sense of positivism.

25. Embrace Vulnerability:

- Allow yourselves to be vulnerable with each other, disclosing anxieties, worries, and hopes.

26. Reminisce and Reflect:

- Reminisce about the situations that brought you together and reflect on the journey you've travelled so far.

27. Practice Mindfulness Together:

- Engage in mindfulness exercises, meditation, or relaxation techniques as a pair to promote a sense of peace.

28. Maintain Social Connections:

- Stay connected with friends and family who provide emotional support and a feeling of normalcy.

29. Incorporate Touch:

- Touch treatment like massages or mild caresses can be calming and reaffirm your emotional connection.

30. Explore New Activities:

- Engage in activities you've never undertaken before, establishing shared experiences that strengthen your friendship.

31. Plan Date Nights:

- Plan special date evenings or activities that allow you to focus on each other beyond the domain of cancer.

32. Write Letters or Journals:

- Write letters or keep journals to discuss your thoughts and feelings, providing an outlet for emotional expression.

33. Focus on Nonverbal Communication:

- Pay attention to nonverbal indications, gestures, and eye contact that express emotions without words.

34. Adapt to Changes:

- As the cancer journey unfolds, adapt your strategies and approaches to maintain intimacy.

35. Honor Each Other's Coping Styles:

- Respect that each of you may cope differently, and encourage each other's coping skills.

36. Learn Together:

- Educate yourselves about cancer, its therapies, and coping methods as a team.

37. Stay Playful:

- Infuse playfulness into your interactions, reminding yourselves of the light moments that make your partnership fantastic.

38. Capture Moments:

- Capture experiences through pictures, films, or keepsakes to treasure memories and emotions shared.

39. Take Breaks:
- Balance the attention on cancer with breaks where you simply enjoy one other's company without addressing the sickness.

40. Cultivate Gratitude:
- Cultivate a sense of thanks for the moments you share together, highlighting the significance of your connection.

Maintaining intimacy and emotional connection during the trials of cancer is an ongoing effort that takes patience, compassion, and dedication.

By embracing these strategies and modifying them to your situation, you may continue to establish your relationship's foundation and grow together during hardships.

Remember that your path is a monument to the power of love, support, and persistence and that you're not alone in battling these challenges. Seek the support of healthcare professionals, counsellors, and support groups to further develop your journey of intimacy and emotional connection.

Chapter 8

COPING STRATEGIES FOR FAMILIES WHEN A LOVED ONE HAS CANCER

When a family member is diagnosed with cancer, it can be a sad and hard experience for everyone concerned.

Coping with the emotional, practical, and psychological implications of the diagnosis demands fortitude, resilience, and support. Here, we cover complete coping alternatives for families surviving the journey of cancer together:

1. Open Communication:
- Create an environment where open debate is encouraged. Share thoughts, feelings, and concerns honestly.

2. Educate Yourselves:

- Learn about the particular type of cancer, treatment choices, potential side effects, and prognosis to make informed decisions.

3. Seek Professional Guidance:

- Consult medical specialists and seek advice from oncologists, nurses, and social workers who specialise in cancer care.

4. Share Responsibilities:

- Distribute caregiving and home responsibilities among family members to prevent burnout.

5. Accept Support:

- Don't hesitate to accept help from friends, extended family, and support groups. Allow folks to aid you.

6. Create a Support Network:

- Build a community of friends, family, and support groups who understand your situation and provide emotional support.

7. Emotional Expression:
- Encourage everyone to communicate their feelings, worries, and anxieties without judgement.

8. Set Realistic Expectations:
- Understand that there will be good and bad days. Set realistic expectations and be kind with yourselves.

9. Maintain Routines:
- Keep a sense of normalcy by following daily routines as much as possible, which can provide stability.

10. Practising Self-Care:
- Prioritise self-care for each family member, ensuring that emotional and physical well-being is nurtured.

11. Offer Flexibility:

- Be flexible in your goals and expectations, adjusting to changes in treatment schedules or individual circumstances.

12. Celebrate Small Victories:

- Acknowledge and celebrate even the tiniest successes and milestones along the road.

13. Encourage Emotional Outlets:

- Encourage creative outlets such as painting, music, writing, or exercise to enable family members cope with emotions.

14. Seek Professional Help:

- Consider family therapy or counselling to manage tough emotions and promote communication.

15. Respecting Individual Coping Styles:

- Understand that each family member might cope differently. Respect these distinctions and provide aid accordingly.

16. Focus on Quality Time:

- Spend precious time together doing activities that give delight and make lovely memories.

17. Explore Mindfulness and Relaxation:

- Practise mindfulness techniques, meditation, or relaxation exercises as a family to reduce stress.

18. Encourage Positive Thinking:

- Focus on good things, preserve hope and encourage each other's outlook on the issue.

19. Address Financial Concerns:

- If applicable, discuss and plan for any financial issues or challenges that might develop.

20. Nurture Bonding:
- Strengthen family bonds through sharing stories, traditions, and experiences that bring you closer together.

21. Encourage Individual Expression:
- Recognize that each family member copes uniquely. Encourage individual expressions of emotions without judgement.

22. Maintain Boundaries:
- Establish clear boundaries between caregiving obligations and personal space to prevent burnout.

23. Foster Empathy:
- Empathise with one another's experiences, acknowledging the issues and feelings each family member confronts.

24. Plan Together:
- Involve the entire family in establishing treatment schedules, appointments, and supportive care routines.

25. Encourage Children's Expression:
- Create a secure environment for children to ask questions, explore feelings, and voice concerns.

26. Embrace Humour:
- Humor can be a useful coping method. Embrace moments of fun and lightness amid the hurdles.

27. Celebrate Uniqueness:
- Celebrate each family member's skills, talents, and contributions to the family unit.

28. Maintain Flexibility:
- Be adaptive to changes in treatment programs, emotional requirements, and unforeseen circumstances.

29. Practice Gratitude:
- Regularly express gratitude for the support and strength your family provides to one another.

30. Create Memory Keepsakes:
- Document the journey using photographs, journal notes, or video diaries to retain memories.

31. Encourage Independence:
- Allow the affected family member to preserve a sense of independence wherever feasible, empowering their decision-making.

32. Focus on Life Beyond Cancer:
- Balance discussions about cancer with chats about interests, aspirations, and ambitions.

33. Involve Children Appropriately:
- Discuss cancer with children in an age-appropriate manner, answering their questions honestly while providing reassurance.

34. Celebrate Family Strength:

- Celebrate your family's tenacity and courage in overcoming issues together.

35. Support Siblings:

- Pay attention to the needs of siblings, offering them opportunities to express their feelings and fears.

36. Create a Safe Space:

- Establish a safe and non-judgmental space where family members can communicate their feelings without fear.

37. Be Mindful of Language:

- Use upbeat words to promote optimism and stimulate debates.

38. Share Information:

- Share vital facts about therapies, side effects, and the cancer journey to create understanding.

39. Express Love Regularly:
- Remind each other of your love and dedication with verbal affirmations and physical gestures.

40. Embrace the Journey:
- Approach the journey as a united family, focussing on the strength and love that ties you together.

Coping with a family member's cancer diagnosis is a collective undertaking that takes patience, understanding, and continual support.

By continuing to embrace these coping methods and personalising them to your family's individual dynamics, you may manage the obstacles with resilience and togetherness.

Remember that your family's capacity to come together on this journey demonstrates the strength of love, compassion, and solidarity. Seek help from healthcare specialists, support groups, and therapy to further enrich your family's journey of coping and healing.

Chapter 9

THE LANDSCAPE OF CANCER TREATMENTS

Cancer treatment is a fast-growing topic that involves a diverse spectrum of treatments aimed at targeting and eliminating cancer cells while avoiding harm to healthy tissues.

These treatments are tailored to the type of cancer, its stage, and the unique patient's health and preferences. Here, we dig into the complexities of several cancer therapeutic modalities, detailing their mechanics, benefits, and potential harmful effects.

SURGERY

Surgery is a cornerstone of cancer treatment, usually utilised to remove tumours and damaged tissues. It might be curative, offering the prospect of complete elimination of cancer, or palliative, aiming at alleviating symptoms and boosting the quality of life.

While surgery provides immense promise, comprehending its benefits and pitfalls is crucial for patients and their healthcare teams to make informed treatment decisions.

Benefits of Surgical Treatment

1. Curative Intent:

- Surgery tries to thoroughly remove malignant tumours or tissues. When successful, it can remove cancer cells from the body, presenting the opportunity for treatment, especially in early-stage cancers.

2. Localised Control:

- Surgery is effective for tumours that are limited to a specific region. It provides focused control by physically removing malignant growths and preventing their spread to neighbouring tissues.

3. Improved Prognosis:

- Surgical removal of cancer at an early stage can lead to improved long-term results and survival rates, depending on the type of cancer and its characteristics.

4. Immediate Results:

- Unlike some other treatment options, surgery delivers immediate results. Patients can watch the actual eradication of the tumour and get relief from related symptoms.

5. Tissue Sample for Diagnosis:

- Surgical procedures often yield a tissue sample (biopsy) for reliable diagnosis, which informs further treatment options.

6. Adjuvant Therapy Enhancement:
- After surgery, adjuvant therapies like chemotherapy or radiation therapy may be more successful, as the tumour load has been reduced.

Risks and Considerations
1. Anaesthesia Risks:
- Anesthesia carries intrinsic hazards, including allergic responses, adverse effects on the cardiovascular system, and respiratory issues.

2. Bleeding and Infection:
- Surgical operations carry a danger of bleeding and infection at the surgical site, which can lead to difficulties.

3. Damage to Surrounding Structures:

- Surgery can mistakenly harm nearby organs, blood arteries, or nerves, resulting in potential functional limits.

4. Scarring and Disfigurement:
- Depending on the site of the treatment, scars and disfigurement can follow, hurting body image and self-esteem.

5. Pain and Discomfort:
- Post-surgical pain is frequent and could vary in degree depending on the scope of the treatment.

6. Recovery Time:
- Surgical rehabilitation can be protracted, prompting patients to take time off work and adjust their typical activities.

7. Need for Additional Treatments:
- Surgery might not be the single treatment required, as some tumours necessitate additional drugs such chemotherapy, radiation, or targeted therapies.

8. Possible Spread of Cancer Cells:

- In some cases, surgical manipulation could mistakenly release cancer cells into the bloodstream or lymphatic system, potentially leading to the spread of cancer.

9. Anaesthetic Considerations:

- Patients with specific medical problems may suffer additional hazards during surgery due to their health status.

Surgery is a potent instrument in the arsenal of cancer treatments, allowing comprehensive excision of tumours and malignant tissues. However, like any medical procedure, surgery comes with inherent dangers and considerations.

The option to pursue surgery should be a collaborative one involving the patient, their healthcare team, and a comprehensive awareness of the potential advantages and dangers.

RADIATION THERAPY

- Radiation therapy uses high-energy rays to target and destroy cancer cells. It can be delivered externally (external beam radiation) or internally (brachytherapy). The goal is to break the DNA within cancer cells, preventing them from multiplying and developing.

Benefits of Radiation Therapy
1. Precise Targeting:
- Radiation therapy can be precisely focused on the tumour or damaged area, limiting damage to neighbouring healthy tissues.

2. Curative Potential:
- For many kinds of cancer, radiation therapy provides a curative potential, especially when coupled with surgery or other treatments.

3. Adjuvant Therapy:

- Radiation can be used as adjuvant therapy after surgery to eliminate any residual cancer cells and minimise the risk of recurrence.

4. Pain and Symptom Management:

- Radiation therapy can successfully relieve pain and other symptoms caused by tumours that are difficult to remove surgically.

5. Non-Invasive Treatment:

- Unlike surgery, radiation therapy is non-invasive and does not require incisions. It's delivered outside or internally.

6. Localised Control:

- Radiation is beneficial for treating restricted tumours, inhibiting their growth and spread in the targeted area.

7. Organ Preservation:

- In instances when surgery can result in the loss of vital organs or functions, radiation therapy might assist in preserving organ function.

8. Outpatient Treatment:
- Most radiation treatments are outpatient procedures, allowing patients to return home afterward.

Risks and Considerations
1. Skin Reactions:
- Skin in the treatment site may become red, irritated, or even blistering, like a sunburn.

2. Fatigue:
- Radiation therapy can add to tiredness, especially as treatment advances. Patients might need to adjust their everyday activities.

3. Damage to Healthy Tissues:

- Although steps are done to shield healthy tissues, radiation can mistakenly destroy neighbouring organs and tissues.

4. Long-Term Side Effects:
- Some side effects, such as fibrosis or scarring, could emerge months or years after therapy.

5. Impact on Organs:
- Radiation near vital organs like the heart or lungs can raise the probability of long-term complications.

6. Radiation Sickness:
- High quantities of radiation can lead to radiation sickness, causing symptoms like nausea, vomiting, and diarrhoea.

7. Risk of Secondary Cancers:

- Radiation exposure raises the risk of having secondary cancers in the treated location, however this risk is typically minimal.

8. Temporary Infertility:
- Radiation therapy targeting the reproductive organs could result in temporary or permanent infertility.

9. Emotional Impact:
- The emotional toll of radiation therapy, notably fear, and worry, should not be underestimated.

Radiation therapy is a formidable tool in the fight against cancer, delivering significant benefits by precisely targeting and killing cancer cells. However, like any medical treatment, it comes with potential hazards and considerations that need to be appropriately assessed.

The option to accept radiation therapy should be taken collectively between the patient and their healthcare team, taking into account the sort and stage of cancer, overall health, and individual preferences.

CHEMOTHERAPY

- Chemotherapy is the use of powerful drugs to kill or slow the growth of cancer cells. It can be given orally, intravenously, or topically.

Chemotherapy targets fast-dividing cells, which includes both cancer cells and some healthy cells, resulting in potential harmful effects.

Chemotherapy, also referred to as "chemo," is a systemic cancer treatment that uses powerful drugs to target and destroy rapidly dividing cancer cells throughout the body.

<u>Benefits of Chemotherapy</u>

1. Systemic Treatment:

- Chemotherapy circulates throughout the body, targeting cancer cells that may have spread beyond the main tumour location.

2. Curative Potential:

- For some malignancies, chemotherapy can offer curative promise, especially when coupled with surgery, radiation therapy, or other treatments.

3. Adjuvant Therapy:

- Chemotherapy can be used as adjuvant therapy after surgery or other therapies to eradicate any residual cancer cells and minimise the risk of recurrence.

4. Shrinking Tumours:

- Chemotherapy can reduce tumours before surgery, making them easier to remove.

5. Palliative Care:

- Chemotherapy can provide palliative care, easing symptoms and enhancing the quality of life for patients with advanced cancer.

6. Variety of Cancer Types:

- Chemotherapy is used to treat several forms of cancer, making it a versatile treatment alternative.

7. Combination Therapies:

- Chemotherapy can be paired with other treatments including targeted medicines and immunotherapy to increase its effectiveness.

8. Nonsurgical Approach:

- Chemotherapy is a nonsurgical method, making it appropriate for patients who cannot undergo surgery.

<u>Risks and Considerations</u>

1. Side Effects:

- Chemotherapy usually causes side effects due to its impact on swiftly dividing healthy cells, leading to symptoms including nausea, vomiting, hair loss, tiredness, and more.

2. Suppressed Immune System:

- Chemotherapy can impair the immune system, increasing the risk of infections.

3. Anaemia and Bleeding:

- Chemotherapy can decrease red blood cell counts, leading to anaemia and an increased risk of bleeding.

4. Long-Term Effects:

- Some undesirable effects can linger long after therapy ceases, harming patients' quality of life.

5. Nausea and Vomiting:

- Nausea and vomiting are frequent adverse effects of chemotherapy, although contemporary medications can help manage them.

6. Hair Loss:

- Many chemotherapy medications cause hair loss, affecting body image and self-esteem.

7. Fatigue:

- Chemotherapy-related fatigue can be catastrophic, limiting routine activities and quality of life.

8. Risk of Secondary Cancers:

- Some chemotherapy drugs boost the risk of having secondary cancers, although this risk is typically minor.

9. Emotional Impact:

- Coping with side effects and treatment-related changes could have emotional ramifications, leading to stress and worry.

Chemotherapy is a cornerstone of cancer treatment, delivering a strategy to systematically target and eliminate cancer cells throughout the body.

However, the benefits of chemotherapy need to be assessed against its potential dangers and unwanted effects. The decision to undergo chemotherapy should be decided collectively between the patient and their healthcare team, considering aspects such as cancer kind, stage, overall health, and individual preferences.

TARGETED THERAPY

- Targeted therapy focuses on specific chemicals or processes involved in cancer growth. These drugs strive to inhibit the signalling that enables cancer cell multiplication, minimising damage to healthy cells.

Targeted therapy is a new method of treating cancer that focuses on identifying and removing certain substances or processes involved in the growth and spread of cancer cells.

Unlike traditional chemotherapy, which affects both healthy and cancerous cells, targeted therapy seeks to selectively target cancer cells, limiting risk to adjacent organs. Delving into its benefits and accompanying hazards is crucial for patients and healthcare providers to make informed treatment decisions.

<u>Benefits of Targeted Therapy</u>

1. Precision Treatment:

- Targeted therapy is tailored to the molecular characteristics of a patient's cancer, enhancing its precision and effectiveness.

2. Reduced Harm to Healthy Cells:

- Targeted therapy's selectivity means it selectively attacks cancer cells, reducing damage to healthy tissues and decreasing undesirable effects.

3. Enhanced Treatment Efficacy:

- By targeting specific molecular targets, tailored medications can have a more dramatic effect on cancer cells, typically leading to improved treatment outcomes.

4. Reduced Chemotherapy Side Effects:

- Targeted therapy may have less severe side effects compared to regular chemotherapy.

5. Combination Possibilities:

- Targeted therapies can be paired with other treatments like chemotherapy or immunotherapy to increase their effectiveness.

6. Overcoming Resistance:

- Some cancers acquire resistance to traditional treatments. Targeted therapy gives an additional option for treating resistant cancer cells.

7. Personalised Approach:

- Targeted therapy takes into account an individual's unique genetic composition and the molecular characteristics of their cancer.

Risks and Considerations

1. Development of Resistance:

- Just like other treatments, cancer cells could develop resistance to targeted therapy over time.

2. Limited Applicability:

- Targeted therapies are effective only for malignancies with specific molecular targets, restricting their utility to a group of patients.

3. High Cost:
- Targeted medicines can be expensive due to the complexity of development and the demand for molecular testing.

4. Side Effects:
- While frequently gentler than chemotherapy, targeted therapies can nevertheless elicit unpleasant effects, including skin reactions, gastrointestinal issues, and tiredness.

5. Potential for Overgrowth of Non-Targeted Cells:
- In rare circumstances, targeted therapy could accidentally increase the proliferation of non-targeted cells, resulting in unwanted adverse effects.

6. Emotional and Psychological Impact:
- Coping with the potential limits of concentrated therapy, especially if it's not

productive, could have emotional implications.

7. Individual Variation:
- Response to targeted therapy varies among patients, and it may not be equally beneficial for everyone.

Targeted therapy has altered cancer treatment by offering a more accurate and effective way to target cancer cells at the molecular level.

While it comes with various benefits, patients and healthcare professionals need to weigh these advantages against the potential hazards and constraints.

The decision to conduct targeted therapy should be founded on comprehensive talks between the patient and their healthcare team, including elements such as cancer sort, molecular characteristics, overall health, and individual preferences.

IMMUNOTHERAPY

Immunotherapy boosts the body's natural immune response to target and eliminates cancer cells. It comprises immune checkpoint inhibitors, cancer vaccines, and adoptive T-cell therapies.

Immunotherapy is a new strategy in treating cancer that harnesses the body's immune system to target and eradicate cancer cells.

Unlike standard medicines, which directly kill cancer cells, immunotherapy increases the body's defences to recognize and eradicate these abnormal cells.

Benefits of Immunotherapy

1. Targeted and Systemic Approach:

- Immunotherapy can target cancer cells throughout the body, enabling a systemic approach to treatment.

2. Enhanced Immune Response:
- Immunotherapy boosts the immune system's ability to recognize and fight cancer cells, perhaps leading to long-lasting benefits.

3. Potential for Long-Term Remission:
- In rare circumstances, immunotherapy can lead to lengthy periods of remission, or even entire elimination of cancer.

4. Reduced Harm to Healthy Tissues:
- Immunotherapy selectively targets cancer cells, sparing healthy tissues and reducing side consequences.

5. Combination Potential:
- Immunotherapy can be paired with other treatments like chemotherapy or targeted therapy to increase their effectiveness.

6. Treatment for Advanced Cancers:
- Immunotherapy gives hope to those with advanced or metastatic cancers, where traditional treatments could have limited impact.

7. Diverse Cancer Types:
- Immunotherapy has shown promise in treating a wide range of cancer types, including melanoma, lung cancer, kidney cancer, and more.

<u>Risks and Considerations</u>
1. Immune-Related Side Effects:
- Immunotherapy can lead to immune-related side effects, known as immune-related adverse events (irAEs), affecting organs and systems in the body.

2. Limited Effectiveness in Some Cases:
- While successful for some patients, not everyone responds identically to immunotherapy, and its effectiveness can

vary based on cancer type and individual features.

3. Development of Resistance:
- Just like other treatments, cancer cells could develop resistance to immunotherapy over time.

4. Potentially Severe Side Effects:
- While generally well-tolerated, some immune-related side effects could be severe and require prompt medical intervention.

5. High Costs:
- Immunotherapy therapies can be expensive due to the sophisticated nature of research and administration.

6. Emotional and Psychological Impact:
- Coping with the potential limitations of immunotherapy, especially if it's not effective, can have emotional ramifications.

7. Individual Variation:

- Response to immunotherapy varies among patients, and not all individuals will have the same degree of benefit.

Immunotherapy has transformed cancer treatment by using the capabilities of the immune system to target and eradicate cancer cells.

While it brings enormous benefits, patients and healthcare professionals must examine the potential hazards and constraints. The option to start immunotherapy should involve comprehensive talks between the patient and their healthcare team, examining issues such as cancer sort, individual health, probable adverse effects, and treatment goals.

HORMONE THERAPY

Hormone therapy is applied for hormone-sensitive malignancies such as breast and prostate cancer. It blocks or interferes with hormones that drive the growth of cancer cells.

Hormone treatment is a specialised therapeutic strategy frequently applied in malignancies that are hormone-sensitive, such as breast and prostate cancers.

This therapy tries to prevent or interfere with hormones that stimulate the growth of cancer cells.

While hormone therapy has shown remarkable success, acknowledging its benefits and potential hazards is crucial for patients and healthcare professionals to make informed treatment decisions.

Benefits of Hormone Therapy

1. Effective for Hormone-Sensitive Cancers:

- Hormone therapy is particularly useful for malignancies that are driven by hormones, such as breast and prostate tumours.

2. Slowing Cancer Growth:

- By interfering with hormone signalling pathways, hormone treatment can slow down or halt the growth of hormone-sensitive cancer cells.

3. Prolonging Remission:

- Hormone therapy can increase the duration of remission or delay illness progression, boosting the quality of life.

4. Adjuvant Therapy:

- Hormone medication is widely used as adjuvant therapy after surgery to minimise the probability of cancer recurrence.

5. Non-Invasive Approach:
- Hormone therapy is a non-invasive treatment option, commonly taken orally as pills.

6. Palliative Care:
- Hormone medication can provide palliative care for advanced cancers, easing symptoms and boosting the quality of life.

<u>Risks and Considerations</u>
1. Hormone Fluctuations and Side Effects:
- Hormone therapy can lead to hormone fluctuations, resulting in side effects such as hot flashes, mood issues, and sexual dysfunction.

2. Long-Term Treatment:
- Some patients may need to continue hormone therapy for longer periods, potentially leading to long-term unfavourable effects.

3. Development of Resistance:

- Cancer cells can develop resistance to hormone therapy over time, rendering the treatment less effective.

4. Limited Applicability:

- Hormone therapy is only useful for hormone-sensitive cancers. It may not be suitable for other cancer types.

5. Risk of Bone Health Issues:

- Hormone therapy, particularly in postmenopausal women, might increase the risk of bone loss and fractures.

6. Emotional and Psychological Impact:

- Coping with the potential ill effects of hormone therapy could have emotional and psychological repercussions.

7. Individual Variation:

- Response to hormone therapy varies among patients, and not all individuals will have the same degree of improvement.

8. Risk of Recurrence:

- While hormone therapy can lower the likelihood of recurrence, it may not totally eradicate it.

Hormone therapy is a targeted and effective strategy in the treatment of hormone-sensitive cancers. While it offers enormous benefits, patients and healthcare professionals must carefully balance these advantages against potential risks and constraints.

The decision to undergo hormone therapy should involve comprehensive talks between the patient and their healthcare team, examining issues such as cancer sort, hormonal condition, individual health, probable bad effects, and treatment goals.

STEM CELL TRANSPLANT

- Stem cell transplant (also known as bone marrow transplant) entails replacing damaged bone marrow with healthy stem cells to restore the body's ability to generate blood cells.

A stem cell transplant, commonly known as a bone marrow transplant, is a specialty therapy option used in some types of cancers to replace damaged or diseased bone marrow with healthy stem cells.

These stem cells can develop into different types of blood cells, offering a renewed opportunity for the body to generate healthy blood cells.

While stem cell transplant has proved outstanding success, recognizing its benefits and potential hazards is vital for patients and healthcare providers when making informed treatment decisions.

<u>Benefits of Stem Cell Transplant</u>

1. Replacement of Diseased Bone Marrow:

- Stem cell transplant allows replacing malignant or damaged bone marrow with healthy stem cells, maybe eradicating cancerous cells.

2. Renewed Blood Cell Production:

- Stem cell transplant fosters the creation of new, healthy blood cells, enhancing total blood cell levels.

3. Treatment for Blood Cancers:

- Stem cell transplant is particularly helpful for treating blood-related cancers such as leukaemia, lymphoma, and multiple myeloma.

4. Prolonging Remission:

- Stem cell transplant can lengthen the duration of remission or delay disease progression, increasing the quality of life.

5. Immune System Reset:

- In some circumstances, stem cell transplant includes replacing the immune system, potentially leading to a better and more effective fight against cancer.

6. Treatment for Non-Cancerous Diseases:

- Stem cell transplant is also used to treat non-cancerous disorders such as aplastic anaemia and some inherited defects.

<u>Risks and Considerations</u>

1. Complications from Intense Treatment:

- The conditioning treatment given before the transplant, which involves high-dose chemotherapy or radiation, can produce severe unwanted effects and complications.

2. Graft-Versus-Host Disease (GVHD):

- In allogeneic transplants (using donor stem cells), the immune cells from the donor can attack the recipient's healthy tissues, leading to GVHD.

3. Immunosuppression:

- Immunosuppressive drugs are often essential to avoid GVHD, increasing the risk of infections and other complications.

4. Risk of Transplant Failure:

- The transplanted stem cells may not engraft successfully, leading to transplant failure.

5. Long-Term Effects:

- Stem cell transplant can have long-term implications on the body, including a potential impact on fertility and the risk of recurrent cancers.

6. Emotional and Psychological Impact:

- Coping with the probable side effects and difficulties of stem cell transplant could have emotional and psychological ramifications.

7. Limited Applicability:

- Stem cell transplant is not suited for all cancer types and patient characteristics, and careful patient selection is important.

8. Risk of Relapse:

- While stem cell transplant can prolong remission, it may not totally minimise the probability of cancer returning.

Stem cell transplant is a potent treatment option for certain types of malignancies and non-cancerous illnesses, presenting an opportunity to replace damaged bone marrow with healthy stem cells.

While it has significant benefits, the possible hazards and constraints must be thoroughly assessed. The option to undertake a stem cell transplant should involve comprehensive conversations between the patient and their healthcare team, examining issues such as cancer sort, overall health, probable complications, and treatment goals.

PRECISION MEDICINE

Precision medicine analyses genetic information from a patient's tumour to alter treatment techniques. It seeks to find genetic abnormalities underlying cancer growth and choose treatments that target those specific mutations.

Precision medicine, commonly known as personalised medicine, is a cutting-edge approach to cancer therapy that tailors medical care to the unique genetic makeup of each patient.

This approach considers individual differences in genes, proteins, and other variables to determine the best effective therapy strategy. While precision medicine has enormous promise, acknowledging its benefits and potential hazards is crucial for patients and healthcare professionals to make informed treatment decisions.

Benefits of Precision Medicine

1. Targeted Treatments:

- Precision medicine allows for the detection of precise genetic abnormalities or alterations causing cancer growth, enabling targeted therapy.

2. Improved Treatment Efficacy:

- By targeting the molecular drivers of cancer, precision medicine can lead to more effective treatment outcomes.

3. Reduced Harm to Healthy Cells:
- Precision medicine decreases the influence on healthy cells, lowering undesirable effects frequently associated with traditional treatments.

4. Personalised Approach:
- Tailoring treatment to an individual's genetic profile increases the likelihood of identifying the most suited and successful drug.

5. Optimised Treatment Selection:
- Precision medicine helps healthcare providers choose the appropriate treatment from the outset, eliminating wasteful trials and blunders.

6. Combination Potential:
- Precision medicine treatments can be coupled with other therapy to increase effectiveness.

<u>Risks and Considerations</u>

1. Limited Applicability:

- Not all tumours have detectable genetic aberrations or markers that can be addressed with precision treatment.

2. Developing Resistance:

- Cancer cells can acquire resistance to specific treatments over time, ultimately lowering the treatment's effectiveness.

3. High Costs:

- Precision medicine drugs can be pricey due to the sophisticated nature of genetic testing and the production of particular pharmaceuticals.

4. Complex Testing:

- Genetic testing to determine applicable treatments might be complex and may not always offer obvious results.

5. Emotional and Psychological Impact:
- The danger of treatment resistance or restricted alternatives can have emotional ramifications for patients.

6. Data Privacy Concerns:
- Precision medicine relies on genetic data, generating concerns about data privacy and security.

7. Individual Variation:
- While precision medicine aims to customise treatment, individual reactions to therapy can still differ.

Precision medicine represents a paradigm shift in cancer therapy, giving a personalised strategy that tackles the specific genetic composition of each patient's condition. While it brings enormous benefits, the possible threats and constraints must be carefully addressed.

The decision to seek precision medicine should involve comprehensive talks between the patient and their healthcare team, assessing elements such as cancer kind, genetic profile, medication alternatives, expected adverse effects, and treatment goals.

RADIOFREQUENCY ABLATION

Radiofrequency ablation involves using heat caused by radio waves to kill cancer cells. It is often applied for malignancies that are tiny and limited.

Radiofrequency ablation (RFA) is a minimally invasive medical procedure used to treat certain types of cancer by applying high-frequency electrical currents to heat and destroy cancerous cells.

While RFA offers a less intrusive option to surgery, acknowledging its benefits and potential hazards is crucial for patients and healthcare professionals when making intelligent treatment decisions.

<u>Benefits of Radiofrequency Ablation</u>
1. Minimally Invasive Approach:
- RFA is a minimally invasive therapy that involves only a tiny incision, minimising the need for significant surgical operations.

2. Targeted Treatment:
- RFA allows for accurate targeting of cancerous sites, limiting injury to neighbouring healthy cells.

3. Outpatient Procedure:
- Many RFA surgeries are completed in an outpatient manner, allowing patients to return home the same day.

4. Quick Recovery Time:
- Compared to traditional surgery, RFA typically results in quicker recovery times and shorter hospital stays.

5. Localised Treatment:
- RFA is successful in treating restricted tumours, making it particularly useful for those who are not candidates for surgery.

6. Palliative Care:
- RFA can be applied to alleviate discomfort and enhance the quality of life in patients with advanced cancers.

7. Combination Therapy:
- RFA can be paired with other treatments including chemotherapy or radiation therapy to increase therapeutic success.

Risks and Considerations
1. Incomplete Ablation:
- In some instances, RFA might not completely destroy all cancer cells, resulting in the probability of cancer recurrence.

2. Risk of Bleeding and Infection:
- RFA methods carry a risk of bleeding and infection at the treatment site.

3. Damage to Nearby Structures:
- There is a potential of harming surrounding blood vessels, nerves, or organs during the treatment.

4. Pain and Discomfort:
- Patients could experience pain, discomfort, or soreness at the treatment site following RFA.

5. Skin Burns:
- Rarely, RFA could lead to skin burns at the insertion point of the electrode.

6. Need for Repeat Procedures:
- Depending on the tumour's characteristics, some patients could require several RFA sessions for best results.

7. Potential Side Effects:

- Some people may have side effects such as fever, infection, or changes in blood pressure.

8. Emotional Impact:

- Coping with the probable repercussions and effects of RFA could have emotional and psychological implications.

Radiofrequency ablation is a minimally invasive therapeutic procedure that holds promise for certain types of cancer, allowing targeted and localised eradication of malignant cells.

However, patients and healthcare providers must carefully assess its benefits and potential dangers. The choice to perform RFA should involve comprehensive conversations between the patient and their healthcare team, examining issues such as cancer kind, tumour location, anticipated repercussions, and treatment goals.

<u>CRYOTHERAPY</u>

Cryotherapy freezes and destroys cancer cells. It is often used for restricted tumours, such as prostate cancer.

Cryotherapy, also known as cryoablation or cryosurgery, is a medical treatment that uses severe cold to destroy malignant or abnormal tissues.

In the context of cancer treatment, cryotherapy involves freezing cancer cells, forcing them to die and be reabsorbed by the body.

While cryotherapy offers a less invasive option to standard surgery, appreciating its benefits and potential hazards is crucial for patients and healthcare providers when choosing treatment possibilities.

<u>**Benefits of Cryotherapy**</u>

1. Minimally Invasive Approach:

- Cryotherapy is minimally invasive, often requiring just tiny incisions or needles to access the treatment region.

2. Precise Targeting:

- Cryotherapy provides precision targeting of malignant tumours, minimising harm to neighbouring healthy cells.

3. Outpatient Procedure:

- Many cryotherapy surgeries are undertaken on an outpatient basis, allowing patients to return home the same day.

4. Quick Recovery Time:

- Compared to normal surgery, cryotherapy typically results in quicker recovery times and shorter hospital stays.

5. Localised Treatment:

- Cryotherapy is helpful for treating localised tumours, making it suitable for those who are not candidates for extensive surgery.

6. Pain Management:
- Cryotherapy can deliver pain relief by numbing nerve endings in the treated area.

7. Palliative Care:
- Cryotherapy can be utilised for palliative treatment in patients with advanced cancers, alleviating discomfort and boosting the quality of life.

8. Combination Therapy:
- Cryotherapy can be paired with other treatments like chemotherapy or radiation therapy to increase therapeutic success.

Risks and Considerations
1. Incomplete Treatment:
- In rare instances, cryotherapy might not entirely eliminate all cancer cells, resulting in the probability of cancer recurrence.

2. Risk of Bleeding and Infection:

- Cryotherapy treatments pose a danger of bleeding and infection at the treatment site.

3. Damage to Nearby Structures:

- There is a risk of injuring surrounding blood vessels, nerves, or organs during the freezing treatment.

4. Nerve Damage:

- Cryotherapy can lead to nerve damage in the treated area, resulting in numbness or loss of sensation.

5. Skin Damage:

- Rarely, cryotherapy can cause skin damage or changes in pigmentation at the treatment site.

6. Need for Repeat Procedures:

- Depending on the tumour's characteristics, some individuals could require several cryotherapy sessions for excellent outcomes.

7. Swelling and Discomfort:
- Patients could endure swelling, discomfort, or pain at the treatment site following cryotherapy.

8. Emotional Impact:
- Coping with the potential complications and outcomes of cryotherapy could have emotional and psychological implications.

Cryotherapy is a minimally invasive treatment strategy that holds promise for certain types of cancer, delivering precise and localised eradication of malignant cells.

However, patients and healthcare providers must carefully assess its benefits and potential dangers. The decision to undertake cryotherapy should involve comprehensive conversations between the patient and their healthcare team, examining issues such as cancer kind, tumour location, potential repercussions, and treatment goals.

PHOTODYNAMIC THERAPY

Photodynamic therapy combines light-sensitive medications and lasers to destroy cancer cells. It's commonly employed for skin malignancies and specific sorts of inner cancers.

Photodynamic treatment (PDT) is a new medical procedure that utilises light-sensitive compounds to specifically target and destroy cancer cells.

By blending light, photosensitizing drugs, and oxygen, PDT offers a new approach to cancer treatment.

While PDT holds immense promise, comprehending its benefits and potential dangers is crucial for patients and healthcare professionals to make informed treatment decisions.

<u>Benefits of Photodynamic Therapy</u>

1. Selective Targeting:

- PDT can specifically target cancer cells while sparing healthy surrounding tissues, decreasing collateral effects.

2. Minimally Invasive:

- PDT is typically minimally invasive, necessitating merely the insertion of light-emitting devices or the administration of photosensitizing medications.

3. Precise Localization:

- Light can be carefully targeted on the treatment area, enabling localised treatment of cancers.

4. Limited Side Effects:

- Compared to traditional medicines, PDT frequently results in less systemic side effects.

5. Outpatient Procedure:

- Many PDT sessions are performed in an outpatient manner, allowing patients to return home the same day.

6. Quick Recovery:

- PDT typically leads to quicker recovery times and shorter hospital stays compared to more invasive procedures.

7. Potential for Repeat Treatment:

- PDT can be conducted several times if necessary, as it doesn't cause cumulative damage to healthy tissues.

8. Combination Potential:

- PDT can be paired with other treatments such surgery, radiation, or chemotherapy to improve its effectiveness.

<u>**Risks and Considerations**</u>

1. Light Sensitivity:
- After administration of photosensitizing medications, patients must avoid exposure to bright light, especially sunshine.

2. Limited Depth of Penetration:
- PDT's effectiveness is limited to regions where light can reach, which may restrict its usage in deeper or larger tumours.

3. Incomplete Treatment:
- PDT may not entirely eliminate all cancer cells, leading to the probability of cancer recurrence.

4. Temporary Side Effects:
- After PDT, patients may experience transient adverse effects such as skin irritation, redness, and edema.

5. Effectiveness Depends on Tumour Type:

- PDT is highly helpful for superficial malignancies and specific kinds of malignancy.

6. Limited Applicability:

- PDT may not be suitable for all cancer types and patient characteristics, and careful patient selection is needed.

7. Emotional and Psychological Impact:

- Coping with the expected constraints and results of PDT could have emotional and psychological implications.

8. Individual Variation:

- Response to PDT varies among patients, and not all individuals will have the same degree of benefit.

Photodynamic therapy is a new and specialised strategy for treating certain types of cancer, having the potential to selectively kill cancer cells while minimising harm to healthy tissues.

However, patients and healthcare providers must carefully assess its benefits and potential dangers.

The decision to perform PDT should involve comprehensive talks with the patient and their healthcare team, assessing issues such as disease kind, tumour location, probable repercussions, and treatment goals.

ANGIOGENESIS INHIBITORS

- Angiogenesis inhibitors impede the formation of new blood vessels that tumours need to grow. By cutting off their blood supply, these drugs help starve cancer cells.

Angiogenesis inhibitors represent a novel approach to cancer treatment that targets the process of angiogenesis - the formation of new blood vessels to deliver nutrition and oxygen to tumours.

These inhibitors act by inhibiting the formation of blood vessels, therefore starving the tumour of its vital supplies. While angiogenesis inhibitors give substantial potential, knowing their advantages and potential hazards is crucial for patients and healthcare providers when choosing therapy alternatives.

<u>Benefits of Angiogenesis Inhibitors</u>

1. Stalling Tumour Growth:

- Angiogenesis inhibitors impede the development of new blood vessels, which can slow down or even prevent tumour growth.

2. Targeting Multiple Cancers:

- Angiogenesis inhibitors have proved success in treating several cancer types, making them a versatile alternative.

3. Prolonging Remission:
- These inhibitors can increase the duration of remission or slow down disease development, boosting patients' quality of life.

4. Enhanced Response to Treatment:
- Angiogenesis inhibitors can increase the efficiency of other treatments like chemotherapy or radiation therapy.

5. Reduced Metastasis:
- By limiting blood vessel development, these inhibitors can restrict the spread of cancer to distant organs.

6. Combination Potential:
- Angiogenesis inhibitors can be taken with other drugs for a synergistic effect.

7. Palliative Care:
- In later stages of cancer, angiogenesis inhibitors can provide palliative care by easing symptoms.

<u>**Risks and Considerations**</u>

1. Risk of Side Effects:

- Angiogenesis inhibitors can produce side effects including hypertension, haemorrhage, and gastrointestinal difficulties.

2. Blood Clotting Risk:

- Some inhibitors increase the chance of blood clots, which can have serious health effects.

3. Cardiovascular Issues:

- Certain angiogenesis inhibitors may lead to cardiovascular complications, including heart failure.

4. Wound Healing Interference:

- These inhibitors can limit the body's capacity to repair wounds correctly.

5. Resistance Development:

- Over time, cancer cells may develop resistance to angiogenesis inhibitors, reducing therapy efficacy.

6. Impact on Normal Blood Vessels:

- Angiogenesis inhibitors may damage regular blood arteries, leading to significant complications.

7. Emotional Impact:

- Coping with probable side effects and limits of angiogenesis inhibitors can have emotional and psychological repercussions.

8. Individual Variation:

- Response to angiogenesis inhibitors could vary among patients, and not everyone will have the same degree of improvement.

Angiogenesis inhibitors constitute a prospective path in cancer treatment by targeting the crucial process of blood vessel formation in malignancies.

However, patients and healthcare providers must carefully examine their benefits and potential risks.

The decision to study angiogenesis inhibitors should involve comprehensive talks between the patient and their healthcare team, examining issues such as cancer sort, possible bad effects, treatment goals, and overall health.

COMBINATION THERAPIES

- Many patients endure a mix of treatments, often called multimodal therapy. This strategy aims to assault cancer cells through several mechanisms, enhancing the likelihood of success.

Combination therapy in cancer treatment comprises the simultaneous or sequential employment of different therapeutic techniques to address the illness from multiple angles. These therapies can comprise a mix of surgery, chemotherapy, radiation therapy, immunotherapy, targeted therapy, and more.

While combination treatments have significant promise for enhanced treatment outcomes, knowing their advantages and potential dangers is crucial for patients and healthcare professionals when considering treatment regimens.

Benefits of Combination Therapies

1. Enhanced Treatment Efficacy:
- Combination drugs assault cancer cells through diverse strategies, often leading to greater therapeutic effectiveness.

2. Synergistic Effects:
- Some therapy options interact synergistically, improving the therapeutic impact on cancer cells.

3. Overcoming Resistance:

- Combination treatments can assist overcome therapeutic resistance that cancer cells could acquire against a single therapy.

4. Targeting Multiple Aspects:

- Different treatments can target distinct parts of cancer progression, from tumour growth to metastasis.

5. Personalised Approach:

- Combination therapy can be adjusted to the unique patient's cancer sort, stage, and genetic profile.

6. Improved Survival Rates:

- Studies have revealed that specific combination therapy can lead to improved long-term survival rates for some malignancies.

7. Reducing Doses:
- Some combination drugs allow for lower doses of individual treatments, lowering the risk of side effects.

Risks and Considerations
1. Increased Side Effects:
- Combining therapies can greatly boost the risk and severity of adverse effects, decreasing patients' quality of life.

2. Complex Treatment Plans:
- Combination drugs generally require careful coordination, monitoring, and management of varied treatment schedules.

3. Cumulative Toxicity:
- Some treatments can have cumulative negative effects on the body when used together over an extended period.

4. Interactions and Complications:

- Different medicines could interact with one another or lead to unanticipated issues.

5. Emotional and Psychological Impact:
- Managing the potential adverse effects and challenges of combination therapy could have emotional repercussions.

6. Individual Variation:
- Response to combination therapy varies among patients, and not all individuals will have the same degree of improvement.

7. Cost and Accessibility:
- Combination therapies can be more expensive and might not be accessible to all patients.

8. Decision Complexity:
- Determining the appropriate combination therapy can be complex, requiring careful consideration of individual features.

Combination therapy in cancer treatment gives a potent way to fight the disease by tackling it through various approaches. However, patients and healthcare providers must carefully examine their benefits and potential risks.

The decision to explore combination therapy should involve comprehensive talks between the patient and their healthcare team, examining issues such as cancer sort, treatment modalities, possible adverse effects, treatment goals, and overall health.

PALLIATIVE CARE

Palliative care focuses on increasing the quality of life for patients by managing symptoms, discomfort, and emotional distress. It can be used alongside curative therapy.

Palliative care is a specific approach to medical care that focuses on providing relief from the symptoms, discomfort, and emotional suffering associated with serious illnesses, including cancer.

It is meant to improve the quality of life for patients and their families by meeting physical, emotional, social, and spiritual concerns. While palliative care delivers critical support, recognizing its benefits and potential hazards is crucial for patients and healthcare workers to deliver thorough treatment.

<u>Benefits of Palliative Care</u>
1. Enhanced Quality of Life:
- Palliative care seeks to alleviate pain and discomfort, leading to an enhanced overall quality of life for patients.

2. Comprehensive Symptom Management:
- Palliative care doctors handle a range of symptoms such as pain, tiredness, nausea,

and shortness of breath, improving patients' comfort.

3. Emotional and Psychological Support:

- Palliative care provides emotional counselling and psychological assistance to help patients and families cope with the sufferings of cancer.

4. Holistic Approach:

- Palliative care takes into account patients' physical, emotional, and spiritual well-being, generating a holistic experience of care.

5. Communication and Decision-Making:

- Palliative care experts encourage discussions about treatment choices, goals of care, and advanced care planning.

6. Caregiver Support:

- Palliative care emphasises the significance of aiding carers, giving resources and knowledge to help them handle their position effectively.

7. Consistent Coordination:

- Palliative care teams work with other medical specialists to enable seamless coordination of treatment.

8. Continuity of Care:

- Palliative care can be administered at any stage of the disease, from diagnosis through treatment and into survivorship or end-of-life care.

Risks and Considerations

1. Misconceptions:

- Some patients and families mistakenly misunderstand palliative care as primarily appropriate for end-of-life situations.

2. Delayed Initiation:
- Palliative care should ideally begin early in the cancer journey, but misconceptions could postpone its initiation.

3. Communication Challenges:
- Discussing palliative care with patients and families can be emotionally taxing and require sensitivity.

4. Cultural and Religious Factors:
- Beliefs and behaviours could influence patients' impressions of palliative care, potentially impacting their acceptance.

5. Emotional and Psychological Impact:
- Accepting palliative treatment could induce emotional and psychological worries about the development of the disease.

6. Uncertain Timing:

- Determining the optimal timing to convert from curative treatment to palliative care can be complex and subjective.

7. Individual Preferences:

- Patients' preferences for the amount of care and treatment choices may differ.

Palliative care performs a key role in extending the quality of life for cancer patients by treating their physical, emotional, and spiritual needs. However, individuals and healthcare professionals must appreciate its benefits and potential hazards.

The decision to embrace palliative care should involve candid discussions between the patient, their family, and healthcare providers.

Cancer treatment is a broad area, containing a multiplicity of approaches that address the intricacy of different cancer forms and stages. The choice of treatment depends on parameters such as the type of cancer, its stage, the patient's overall health, and their preferences.

Advances in research continue to lead to new treatment choices and breakthrough pharmaceuticals that give hope for improved outcomes and enhanced quality of life for those confronting a cancer diagnosis.

Chapter 10

SELF-CARE TECHNIQUES FOR YOURSELF WHEN A LOVED ONE HAS CANCER

Caring for a loved one with cancer can be emotionally and physically exhausting. While offering assistance is necessary, it's also important to focus on your own well-being through self-care.

By engaging in self-care activities, you may preserve your resilience, emotional health, and overall well-being throughout this hard time. Here, we go into thorough self-care practices geared to caregivers and family members:

1. Prioritise Physical Health:
- Maintain a balanced diet, remain hydrated, and engage in regular exercise to increase your physical well-being.

2. Restful Sleep:

- Ensure you receive proper sleep to refresh your body and mind. Establish a bedtime routine for greater sleep quality.

3. Deep Breathing and Meditation:

- Practise deep breathing exercises or meditation to alleviate tension, anxiety, and promote relaxation.

4. Establish Boundaries:

- Set clear boundaries between caregiving obligations and personal time to prevent burnout.

5. Engage in Hobbies:

- Dedicate time to hobbies you enjoy, whether it's reading, gardening, painting, or any creative outlet.

6. Stay Socially Connected:

- Maintain ties with friends and family members to prevent loneliness and receive emotional support.

7. Seek Emotional Outlet:

- Express your feelings through journaling, art, music, or conversing with a trusted friend.

8. Practice Gratitude:

- Focus on the positive aspects of your life and the moments of delight amidst the hardships.

9. Professional Counselling:

- Consider therapy or counselling to examine your emotions and gain advice in managing caregiver stress.

10. Mindful Moments:

- Integrate mindfulness into your day, pausing to appreciate small moments of quiet and presence.

11. Pamper Yourself:

- Treat yourself to a spa day, a relaxing bath, or any self-care activity that makes you feel renewed.

12. Laughter Therapy:

- Watch a hilarious movie, read a humorous book, or engage in activities that elicit laughter.

13. Music and Nature:

- Listen to relaxing music or spend time in nature to raise your mood and relieve tension.

14. Breathing in Nature:

- Take a walk in a park, along the beach, or in the woods to connect with nature and breathe in fresh air.

15. Digital Detox:

- Limit screen time and take breaks from technology to disengage and lessen brain clutter.

16. Express Emotions:

- Allow yourself to cry, vent, or express any feelings without judgement. It's a healthy release.

17. Learn to Say No:

- Don't overcommit yourself. Learn to say no to more obligations when needed.

18. Stay Informed:

- Educate yourself on your loved one's disease, treatment choices, and accessible services.

19. Mindful Nutrition:

- Consume a balanced diet that nourishes your body and boosts your energy levels.

20. Practice Patience:
- Be gentle with yourself and realise that it's okay to feel a range of emotions.

21. Mindful Movement:
- Engage in mild exercises like yoga, tai chi, or strolling to enhance physical and mental wellness.

22. Reflective Journaling:
- Keep a journal to track your ideas, emotions, and progress. Reflecting can be cathartic.

23. Practising Self-Compassion:
- Be kind and compassionate with yourself, understanding that caring is tough and you're trying your best.

24. Attend Support Groups:
- Connect with others who are in similar caring positions. Support groups provide understanding and fellowship.

25. Creative Expression:

- Engage in creative pursuits like writing, drawing, or crafts to channel your feelings and find consolation.

26. Digital Support:

- Join online forums or social media groups where caregivers exchange stories, advice, and encouragement.

27. Time Outdoors:

- Spend time outdoors, whether it's a leisurely stroll, a hike, or sitting in a park to bond with nature.

28. Delegate and Accept Help:

- Don't hesitate to delegate duties and accept aid from others. It's a sign of strength, not weakness.

29. Professional Respite:

- Arrange for professional respite care to take breaks from caregiving and recharge.

30. Mindful Eating:

- Eat consciously, appreciating your meals and choosing wholesome foods that support your well-being.

31. Visualization & Guided Imagery:

- Practice visualisation techniques or listen to guided imagery sessions for relaxation and mental clarity.

32. Self-Care Rituals:

- Create daily self-care rituals, whether it's morning meditation, an evening bath, or a cup of herbal tea.

33. Practice Patience:

- Recognize that caregiving is a journey with ups and downs. Be patient with oneself throughout hard circumstances.

34. Creative Cooking:

- Experiment with cooking new recipes or producing comforting meals that bring you delight.

35. Practise Mindful Listening:

- Listen to soothing music or peaceful noises to alleviate stress and encourage relaxation.

36. Cultivate Resilience:

- Embrace setbacks as opportunities to learn and strengthen your resilience.

37. Mindful Technology Use:

- Use technology mindfully, engaging in activities that offer you joy and avoiding negativity.

38. Volunteer and Give Back:

- Participate in voluntary activities or contribute to a cause you care about, establishing a sense of purpose.

39. Practice Forgiveness:

- Forgive yourself for any perceived failings and remember that self-care is an ongoing process.

40. Celebrate Your Efforts:

- Acknowledge and praise your caring efforts and the great influence you're making.

Caring and for a loved one with cancer is quite a noble journey, but remember that taking care of oneself is a crucial component of this responsibility.

By continuing to adopt these self-care strategies and adapting them to your changing circumstances, you can manage the difficulties of caregiving while maintaining your own well-being.

Prioritising self-care isn't just helpful for you; it also ensures that you can provide the finest care and support to your loved one. As you embrace self-care, you contribute to your own resilience and strength, helping you to confront the obstacles with grace and compassion.

Chapter 11

<u>WHEN THE CANCER IS TERMINAL</u>

When a loved one suffers a serious illness like cancer, it's usual to go through an emotional experience akin to mourning. If the condition is terminal, it's vital to talk about death and plan for the end of life. Yes I realise it can be difficult and even upsetting, but there are strategies to make them easier for both you and your loved one.

Time appears to freeze when you learn that someone you love has a life-threatening illness. Maybe you automatically brushed the news away. Or perhaps you cried or swung into action. No of what transpired that day, time, and life move on after the diagnosis is made—regardless of whether you feel ready to deal.

You and your loved one may have examined promising treatments and possibly had a break from encroaching disease. At some point, though, the sickness may develop terminal, and gradually the end draws nigh. Once future treatments are unlikely to be successful, there is a great deal you can do to mobilise support for both of you.

Some of the aid you need is emotional. The fears and thoughts that come now are better acknowledged than ignored. Some of the support you need addresses practical things.

End-of-life care needs to be organised and funeral plans need to be considered. Legal and financial matters must be addressed now or in the days after the death. This chapter can assist lead you through some of these steps and uncover additional sources of support for you to draw on.

Dealing with anticipatory grief

Often, people sense anticipatory grief when they know someone they care about is critically ill. Anticipatory grief requires grappling with and grieving a loss before it totally occurs.

When someone has a serious illness, there are numerous losses to grieve even before the individual becomes terminally ill—for the person who is dying as well as for their family and friends.

Blows to independence and security, decreased capacities, and restricted ideas of the future are only a few examples of the sad losses people experience.

Just as with sorrow following a death, family, and friends may feel a spectrum of diverse emotions as they adjust to the shifting terrain of their existence. Typical feelings at this time include:

- Sorrow.

- Anxiety.
- Anger.
- Acceptance.
- Depression.
- Denial.

Depending on the nature of the condition and the relationship you share, you may feel closer and more motivated to make the time you have left count.

Perhaps you are immensely anxious about what's to come or so entirely focused on last-resort therapy that you continue to drive away any thoughts of the end. Possibly you desire to release or feel guilty and conflicted.

Although not everyone experiences anticipatory grieving, all of these sentiments are natural for those who do. You may find the following steps comforting:

Talk with sympathetic friends or family members, especially those who have encountered analogous circumstances.

- Join a support group online or in person.

- Read novels or listen to audio intended for carers.

Making Time to Say Goodbye

Although unpleasant in so many ways, terminal sickness provides you time to say "I love you," to share your appreciation and to make amends when necessary. When death strikes unexpectedly, people typically lament not having had an opportunity to complete these tasks.

Sometimes, dying people hold on to life because they think that others aren't ready to let them go. Tell your loved one it's entirely alright to let go when they're ready to do so. The certainty that you will be able to keep on—perhaps to support children to mature or to fulfil another joint dream—may give enormous peace.

How to talk about death

Talking about death is frequently difficult. Possibly you fear that you'll undercut your spouse's will to endure or flood your pal in terror.

Speaking about death may feel like a type of abandonment as it suggests you've given up on the remaining chance of a cure. Your own anxiety, misery, and pain may make the words choke your throat.

But clinicians who care with patients with a terminal illness point out the following:

Some crave reassurance. Some persons towards the end of life are relieved by the sense that they will be cherished, not abandoned, no matter what occurs.

Some wish to chat. They may tire of keeping up a beautiful front or talking around a problem that looms so enormous that every other conversation strikes false notes.

Some are afraid—and seek empathy. They may be masking their own various fears: abandoning loved ones, losing control, being a burden, and leaving tasks and plans undone.

Many people dread a terrible death or the mirrored anxieties of others. Sharing such fears and voicing ideas about dying can help people feel less overwhelmed and alone. It can also alleviate bodily discomfort, which is heightened by dread.

Approaching this hard conversation
Clearly, not everyone who is terminally sick is ready to talk about death. So how will you know when to talk and what to say? Below are some words that may help you. Your role

at this difficult moment is only to open the door to this conversation and vow to stay for it if the person you care for desires to talk.

Look for openings

A sermon or song you heard, a book you read, or the way someone else's illness and death progressed can be an occasion for words that open the door. By commenting, you show that you're willing to discuss and needn't be protected.

Seek spiritual advice

Talk with your religious leader or counsellor. Priests, rabbis, and other religious leaders can bring immense solace to believers. Even people who do not routinely attend religious services may turn toward their faith when an illness worsens.

Ask for guidance regarding hospice

Hospice specialists and hospital social workers can also help you and the individual who is ill battling with the anxieties surrounding dying. Even if you have elected not to employ a comprehensive range of hospice care, some options are generally available.

Ask a doctor to assist

A doctor's comfort on how physical symptoms would emerge and how pain would be managed can be important. Some doctors can ask gently about fears, as well.

Realise, though, that it's not unusual for doctors (and nurses) to shy away from talking about death. Some feel motivated to do everything and view death as a failure. Being human, they have their own anxieties and pains to reckon with, too.

Let it go

I noticed that people drift into and out of denial during the course of the disease and even during a single session.

Sometimes it's too hard to consider or talk about death. Let your loved one quit conversations that feel too difficult. Allow them to cling to soothing beliefs and illusions.

Chapter 12

<u>COPING AND DEALING WITH THE LOSS OF A LOVED ONE TO CANCER</u>

Losing a loved one to cancer is a profound and sad experience that can significantly touch every aspect of your life.

sorrow is a natural response to this loss, and while the road through sorrow is individually individualised, there are tools and insights that can help you manage this tough time. Here, we cover fully the process of coping and dealing with the loss of a loved one to cancer:

Grief is a complex and personalised process that covers a range of emotions, thoughts, and bodily experiences. It is not a linear journey, and each person's experience is unique.

Grief can emerge as sadness, rage, guilt, bewilderment, and even moments of relief. Acknowledging and allowing these feelings to surface is a vital step toward healing.

Give Yourself Permission to Grieve

Grant yourself permission to grieve in your own way and on your own timing. Understand that there is no "right" way to grieve, and emotions may ebb and go.

Seek Support

Reach out to friends, relatives, support groups, or a professional who specialises in bereavement counselling. Sharing your feelings with those who understand can bring comfort and validation.

Express Your Emotions

Find healthy outlets to vent your feelings. Cry, journal, create art, or participate in activities that allow you to process your feelings.

Practice Self-Compassion

Be compassionate to yourself during this tough period. Treat yourself with the same kindness and empathy you would offer a friend.

Create Meaningful Rituals

Develop routines that commemorate your loved one's memory. Lighting a light, creating a memorial scrapbook, or visiting a particular spot can give solace.

Embrace Memories

Celebrate the pleasant memories and moments spent with your loved one. Focus on their lives rather than exclusively on their passing.

Take Care of Your Physical Health

Grieving can take a toll on your physical well-being. Prioritise sleep, keep a healthy diet, and engage in light exercise to support your body.

Allow Yourself to Heal

Healing doesn't imply forgetting; it means finding a way to carry the memories of your loved one on without being overwhelmed by pain.

Navigating Anniversaries and Triggers

Birthdays, anniversaries, and certain places or objects can evoke significant emotions. Be prepared for these occasions and arrange self-care measures.

Practice Patience

Grief doesn't have a predetermined timeline. Give yourself permission to heal at your own time and don't rush the process.

Honour Your Feelings

Every emotion you experience is valid. It's common to have a mix of sensations, including times of rage, grief, and even joy.

Counselling and Therapy

If your sorrow gets overwhelming, consider obtaining professional treatment from a grief counsellor or therapist to help you negotiate your feelings.

Rediscover Meaning and Purpose

Over time, examine how you can rediscover a feeling of meaning and purpose in your life. This could involve volunteering, following hobbies, or helping those who are mourning.

Remember Self-Care

Continue practising self-care even as you grieve. Taking care of your mental and physical well-being remains vital.

Celebrate Life

In time, as you heal, discover methods to commemorate the life of your loved one. Share memories, make tributes, and keep their legacy alive.

Create a Grief Ritual

Establish a routine that allows you to connect with your loved one's memory. This could involve lighting a candle, planting a tree, or making a donation in their name.

Allow for Triggers

Understand that some sights, sounds, or experiences may evoke overwhelming emotions. It's acceptable to feel these emotions and allow yourself to process them.

Celebrate Their Legacy

Channel your grief into honouring the influence your loved one had on your life and others. Share their tales, achievements, and attributes that made them exceptional.

Join a Support Group

Connecting with people who have endured similar loss can bring a sense of understanding and belonging.

Write a Letter

Write a letter to your loved one explaining your feelings, recollections, and the things you wish you could have said.

Celebrate Special Days

On anniversaries, birthdays, and other key days, commemorate your loved one's life by partaking in activities that honour their memory.

Channel Grief into Creativity

Engage in creative pursuits like writing, painting, or creating to express your emotions and discover a conduit for healing.

Practice Forgiveness

Forgive yourself for any regrets or unresolved sentiments you may have. Letting go of guilt is part of the healing process.

Create a Memory Box

Compile items that remind you of your loved one, such as photos, letters, and souvenirs, in a memory box.

Explore Nature for Solace

Spending time in nature can give peace and allow for calm reflection.

Support Others Grieving

Helping those who are grieving can provide a sense of purpose and link you with the wider community.

Mindfulness and Meditation

Engage in mindfulness and meditation activities to anchor yourself and find moments of quiet among the tempest of emotions.

Celebrate Small Steps

Recognize and celebrate the modest steps you take toward healing. Each step is a testimonial to your strength.

Journal for Healing

Journaling can be a therapeutic outlet for expressing your emotions and recording your journey through loss.

Give Yourself Grace

Grief is not a linear process. There will be good days and bad days. Give yourself grace throughout the hard situations.

Engage in Acts of Kindness

Perform acts of kindness in memory of your loved one, spreading optimism in their name.

Remember Self-Care

Even while you move through your loss, continue prioritising your well-being through self-care activities.

Coping with the loss of a loved one to cancer is a journey that unfolds over time.

Remember that healing is not about forgetting or moving on, but about integrating the memories and emotions into your life in a way that allows you to move forward with renewed purpose and meaning.

By accepting these coping tactics and allowing yourself to grieve authentically, you are respecting your loved one's memory and taking steps toward healing your heart.

As you traverse this path, remember that seeking professional support and relying on the affection of friends and family can be significant sources of comfort and strength.

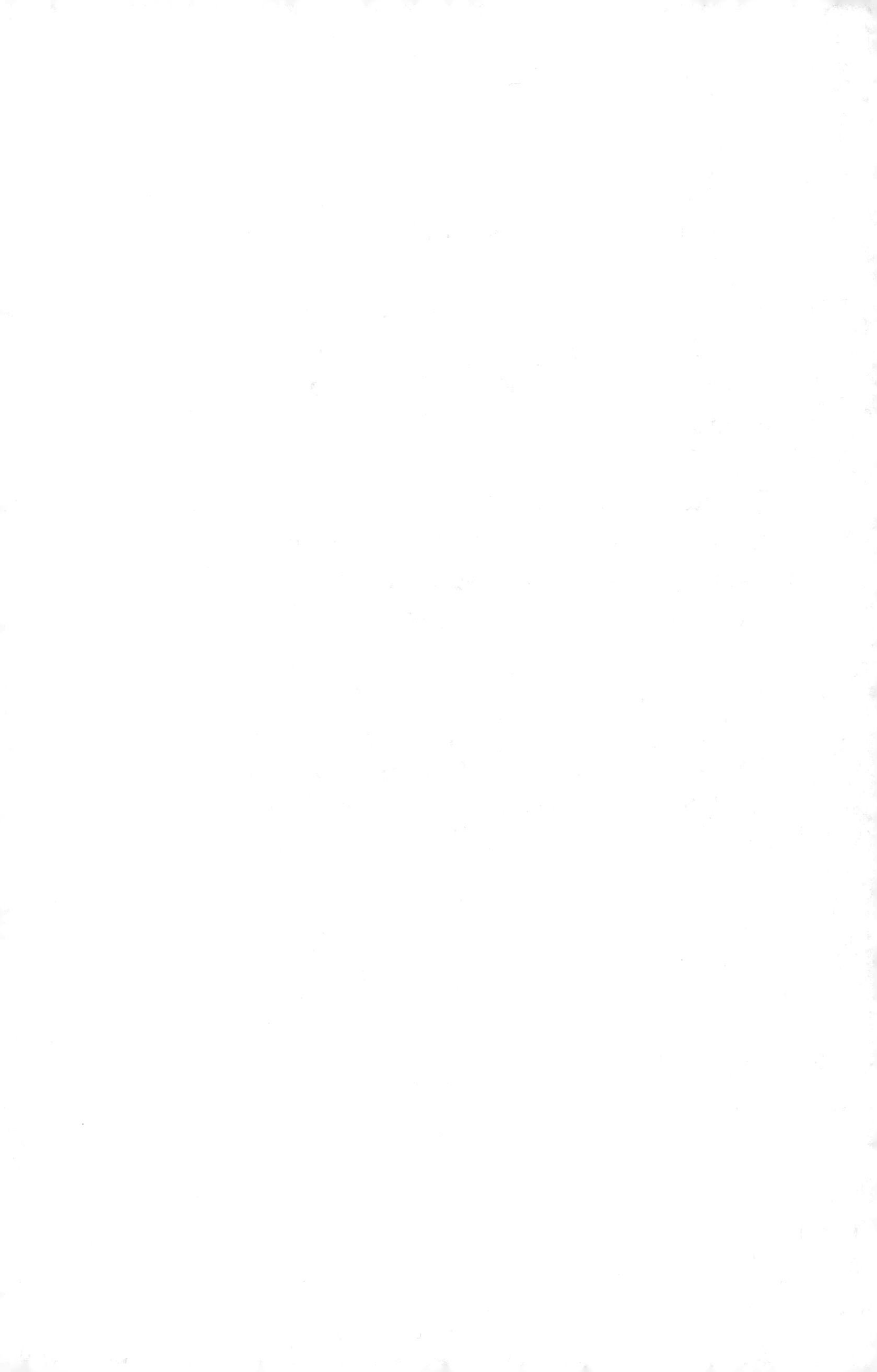